The Pituitary Gland - An Overview of Pathophysiology and Current Management Techniques

Edited by Maleeha Ahmad

Published in London, United Kingdom

The Pituitary Gland - An Overview of Pathophysiology and Current Management Techniques
http://dx.doi.org/10.5772/intechopen.1001527
Edited by Maleeha Ahmad

Contributors
Maleeha Ahmad, Robert J. Weil, Vyacheslav S. Pronin, Mikhail B. Antsiferov, Tatyana M. Alekseeva, Evgeny V. Pronin, Vikram Chakravarthy, Vadim Gospodarev, Jorrdan Bissell, Brandon Edelbach, Timothy Marc Eastin, Kenneth De Los Reyes, Eniola Risikat Kadir, Abdulmalik Omogbolahan Hussein, Lekan Sheriff Ojulari, Gabriel O. Omotoso, Nilima Dongre

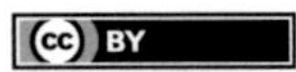

Notice

Statements and opinions expressed in the chapters are these of the individual contributors and not necessarily those of the editors or publisher. No responsibility is accepted for the accuracy of information contained in the published chapters. The publisher assumes no responsibility for any damage or injury to persons or property arising out of the use of any materials, instructions, methods or ideas contained in the book.

First published in London, United Kingdom, 2023 by IntechOpen
IntechOpen is the global imprint of INTECHOPEN LIMITED, registered in England and Wales, registration number: 11086078, 5 Princes Gate Court, London, SW7 2QJ, United Kingdom

British Library Cataloguing-in-Publication Data
A catalogue record for this book is available from the British Library

Additional hard and PDF copies can be obtained from orders@intechopen.com

The Pituitary Gland - An Overview of Pathophysiology and Current Management Techniques
Edited by Maleeha Ahmad
p. cm.
Print ISBN 978-1-83769-565-2
Online ISBN 978-1-83769-564-5
eBook (PDF) ISBN 978-1-83769-566-9

For EU product safety concerns:
IN TECH d.o.o., Prolaz Marije Krucifikse Kozulić 3, 51000 Rijeka, Croatia,
info@intechopen.com or visit our website at intechopen.com.

Meet the editor

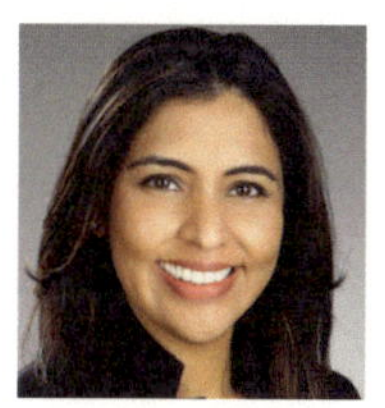

Dr. Ahmad is a distinguished transatlantic neurosurgeon renowned for her expertise in various facets of neurosurgery, including general neurosurgery, the treatment of brain and spinal tumors, and the practice of stereotactic radiosurgery. She holds the esteemed title of fellow at both the Royal College of Surgeons of the United Kingdom and the American College of Surgeons. Dr. Ahmad's academic journey began at the University of Southampton School of Medicine, England, where she graduated with distinction. She subsequently completed her neurosurgical residency with the Yorkshire and Humber School of Surgery, England. Following this, she further honed her skills through a Skull Base and Neurosurgical Oncology Fellowship at Weill Cornell Medical Center and Geisinger Health Systems, USA. Her expertise expanded with specialized training in stereotactic radiosurgery at Stanford University, USA. Not only is Dr. Ahmad a distinguished practitioner, but she is also the author of neurosurgical textbooks. She holds prominent editorial positions with international neurosurgical journals, showcasing her dedication to advancing the field. Dr. Ahmad has spearheaded collaborative academic initiatives and clinical trials on global, regional, and hospital levels, contributing significantly to the neurosurgical community. In her current role as a faculty member at Loma Linda University Health Systems, USA, Dr. Ahmad continues to incorporate cutting-edge technology, including elements of artificial intelligence, and embraces hybrid surgical approaches to further enhance her neurosurgical practice and clinical expertise.

Contents

Preface **IX**

Section 1
Management of Acromegaly **1**

Chapter 1 **3**
Acromegaly: Overview and Current Management Options
by Maleeha Ahmad and Robert J. Weil

Chapter 2 **25**
Using a Precision Approach to Optimize the Drug Therapy of Patients with Acromegaly Syndrome
by Vyacheslav S. Pronin, Mikhail B. Antsiferov, Tatyana M. Alekseeva and Evgeny V. Pronin

Section 2
Operative Nuances in Pituitary Surgery **45**

Chapter 3 **47**
Diaphragma Sellotomy: A Safe Technique to Confirm Adequate Decompression of Optic Chiasm
by Vikram Chakravarthy, Vadim Gospodarev, Jorrdan Bissell, Brandon Edelbach, Timothy Marc Eastin and Kenneth De Los Reyes

Section 3
Role of Pituitary Gland in Reproductive Medicine **57**

Chapter 4 **59**
Role of Pituitary Gland in Fertility Preservation
by Eniola Risikat Kadir, Abdulmalik Omogbolahan Hussein, Lekan Sheriff Ojulari and Gabriel O. Omotoso

Section 4
Complementary Therapies for Pituitary Stimulation **73**

Chapter 5 **75**
Perspective Chapter: Stimulation and Activation of the Pituitary Gland
by Nilima Dongre

Preface

This book is a culmination of expertise contributed by specialists and experts from a wide spectrum of medical fields. It serves as a testament to the profound impact of pituitary diseases, which transcend across various medical disciplines.

The first chapter, "Acromegaly: Overview and Current Management Options" of the book delves deeply into the management of acromegaly, providing an overview of epidemiology, comorbidities, and management algorithms in line with the latest treatment guidelines. In Chapter 2, "Using a Precision Approach to Optimize the Drug Therapy of Patients With Acromegaly Syndrome", Dr. Pronin and colleagues offer a comprehensive insight into the precision-based management techniques currently in use.

In Chapter 3, "Diaphragma Sellotomy: A Safe Technique to Confirm Adequate Decompression of the Optic Chiasm", our respected neurosurgery colleagues, including Dr. Chakravarthy, Dr. Gospodarev, and others, shed light on the intricacies of diaphragma sellotomy. This chapter serves as a comprehensive guide for addressing pituitary adenomas during surgery, catering to both surgical and non-surgical practitioners.

In Chapter 4, "Role of the Pituitary Gland in Fertility Preservation", Dr. Kadir et al. underscore the critical importance of understanding pathways for preserving patients' fertility. It is a valuable resource for healthcare providers.

In Chapter 5, "Perspective Chapter:Stimulation and Activation of the Pituitary Gland", Dr. Dongre offers a fresh and complementary viewpoint, enriching this edition with invaluable insights.

I would like to express my deep appreciation to the chapter authors and the staff at IntechOpen for their invaluable contributions. To you, our esteemed readers, I extend my sincere gratitude for your unwavering commitment to the pursuit of knowledge and your dedication to staying updated in this ever-evolving field of medicine.

With warm regards,

Maleeha Ahmad, MD FRCS (SN) FACS
Department of Neurosurgery,
Loma Linda University Health,
Loma Linda, California, USA

Section 1

Management of Acromegaly

Chapter 1

Acromegaly: Overview and Current Management Options

Maleeha Ahmad and Robert J. Weil

Abstract

Growth-hormone-producing pituitary adenomas in adults will be the focus of this review acromegaly is a disorder caused by pathologically excess levels of growth hormone (GH), nearly always secondary to a pituitary somatotroph adenoma, which account for 10–20% of all pituitary adenomas. Acromegaly is a pan-systemic disease, including but not limited to effects of excess growth hormone on the cardiovascular, respiratory, gastrointestinal, metabolic, and reproductive systems. This raises the concern for clinicians and patients alike in diagnosing the underlying disease when multiple systems are involved. Numerous organ systems may be differentially affected, and the multiplicity of signs and symptoms possibly overlap with other conditions, with the typically slow progression of the disease, it may take years from the initiation of biochemical GH excess before a diagnosis of acromegaly is made. The goal of effective treatment of acromegaly is to eliminate hypersecretion of GH and normalize the production of IGF-1 while preserving normal pituitary function. Medication, radiotherapy, and surgery, often in combination, and over time, are required to mitigate, reduce, and eliminate the morbidity and excess, premature mortality caused by GH elevation.

Keywords: pituitary, adenoma, growth hormone, insulin-like growth factor 1, surgery, medication, radiation, radiosurgery, somatostatin ligand receptors, growth hormone receptor antagonists, dopamine agonists

1. Introduction

Acromegaly, constructed from the Ancient Greek, ακρον, meaning higher, extreme, or tip, and μεγας, for large or bigger, is an uncommon disorder, with an annual incidence in most countries of roughly 5 cases per million population per year. Due to the insidious nature of the signs and symptoms in patients with acromegaly, the overlap of some features, such as weight gain, hypertension, obesity, arthropathies, glucose intolerance, and metabolic syndrome with other, more common disorders, is felt that the true incidence may be higher. Because of this, the prevalence of acromegaly is thought to be underestimated, with figures ranging from 40 to 130 million cases globally [1]. Based on 2010 regional referral practices in the United Kingdom, Brazil, and Belgium, the prevalence of acromegaly may be as high as 400–1000 individuals per million [2].

IntechOpen

2. Pathogenesis

In brief, acromegaly is caused by abnormally elevated levels of growth hormone (GH), which stimulates the synthesis and excess production of insulin-like growth factor 1 (IGF-1), principally from the liver, the small intestines, and within the bones and other tissues in an autocrine/paracrine loop [3, 4].

Under normal conditions, the production and secretion of GH by somatomammotroph cells in the anterior pituitary gland are balanced by stimulatory and inhibitory factors. Growth hormone-releasing hormone (GHRH), produced in the arcuate nucleus of the hypothalamus, is a 44 amino acid peptide that is carried via the hypothalamic-hypophysial portal circulation to the anterior pituitary, where it binds the GHRH receptor and stimulates GH production [5]. GH, a 191 amino acid protein, with a circulatory half-life of several hours, is produced in surges and secreted in a pulsatile manner into the circulation throughout the day and night in a non-circadian pattern, at 3–5 hour intervals [6]. Age, gender, diet, exercise, stress, and other hormones affect GH secretion. Nadirs and zeniths in circulating GH levels may be above or below normal age- and sex-adjusted ranges in both normal patients and those with acromegaly [7].

GH interacts with a cell-surface receptor, the GHR, located in liver, fat, and muscle. Activation of the GHR induces synthesis and secretion of IGF-1 into the systemic circulation [8]. IGF-1 can be produced in local tissues, such as bone, in an autocrine/paracrine fashion. IGF-1 is a 70 amino acid protein with 3 intramolecular sulfide links; in the bloodstream, 98% of IGF-1 is bound to one of six binding proteins (IGF-BPs), which increases IGF-1's stable and effective half-life, on the order of days to weeks. IGF-1 binds the IGF-1 and insulin receptors, more effectively to the former. IGF-1 receptors are found on cells in skeletal and cardiac muscle, bone, cartilage, kidneys, liver, lung, nerves, skin, and hematopoietic system cells. This explains the myriad effects of the GH system [2, 9, 10].

Negative feedback (inhibition) of the GHRH-GH-IGF-1 axis occurs locally, via somatostatin receptor ligand inhibition, as well as systemically, via elevated levels of IGF-1, which act to decrease GH secretion from somatomammotrophs in the anterior pituitary. In the setting of a GH-secreting adenoma, this negative inhibition is muted or absent. This is discussed in detail in the review by Melmed [8].

There are three ways in which acromegaly may result: primary, extra-pituitary, and excess GHRH [10]. Extra-pituitary GH excess is exceptionally uncommon, seen in rare patients with GH-producing abdominal or pancreatic islet tumors. Iatrogenic administration of GH in excess can be seen. Sustained, pathological elevations of GHRH have been reported in patients with a hypothalamic tumor (e.g., a hamartoma) or a peripheral (non-CNS) neuro-endocrine lesion such as a bronchial carcinoid, small cell lung cancer, or adrenal tumors or thyroid medullary cancers. All these conditions are rare and likely require specialist referral and evaluation, over time.

For this review, however, we will concentrate on approximately 95% of patients in whom acromegaly is caused by an adenoma of the anterior pituitary gland.

3. Pathology of pituitary adenoma formation

3.1 General aspects

Pituitary adenomas are benign tumors that are monoclonal in origin and arise from a lineage of differentiated anterior pituitary cells, including gonadotrophs, corticotrophs, thryotrophs, and somatomammotrophs [8, 11]. In the general population, 5–10% of patients may have an adenoma that can be seen on sellar magnetic resonance (MR) imaging, which has a resolution of roughly 1–3 mm; most of these small tumors do not secrete excess hormone and are called incidentalomas [12, 13]. Tumors less than 10 mm are called microadenomas; tumors bigger than 10 mm are macroadenomas. Somewhere between 0.5 and 2% of the population, increasing with increasing age may have a macroadenoma [13, 14]. Tumors may or may not secrete excess levels of hormone; other tumors may not secrete but do produce hormone within the tumor cells, as revealed by immunohistochemical staining. Non-functional and/or non-secretory tumors are more common than adenomas that secrete hormones, namely GH (acromegaly), adrenocorticotropin-secreting hormone (ACTH), thyroid-stimulating hormone (TSH), or prolactin. Of the latter, prolactinomas are the most common, about 20–30% of all patients with a symptomatic adenoma; while ACTH- and GH-secreting adenomas represent 5–10% of patients. Mixed GH and PRL-secreting adenomas are possible, as well.

3.2 What are the histopathological subtypes of somatotroph adenomas?

Pure-growth hormone-secreting adenomas are divided into two subtypes: densely granulated growth hormone [DGGH] cell adenoma and sparsely granulated growth hormone [SGGH] cell adenoma. There is a key difference between these two adenoma sub-types: whilst there is no difference in survival or cure rate, SGGH cell adenomas are more likely to exhibit locally invasive behaviors [15].

Additionally, GH adenomas may also express prolactin in up to half of a surgical series undertaken, when assessed with immunohistochemical staining [15, 16]. One may subdivide tumor types into mixed GH cell/prolactin cell adenoma, mammosomatroph cell adenoma, and acidophilic stem cell adenoma. In approximately a quarter of acromegalic patients, prolactin is also secreted, and elevated levels are measured in the circulation [17].

3.3 What genetic factors are of importance in acromegaly?

GH-secreting adenomas arise as a consequence of unrestrained somatotroph tumor cell proliferation, with multiple defects, including intrinsic cell-cycle dysfunction, altered autocrine and paracrine factors that influence GH synthesis, and cell growth, see **Table 1**. Most GH-secreting adenomas arise sporadically and may or may not have somatic genetic alterations. The most common genetic mutation in sporadic GH-secreting adenomas is a dominant (oncogenic) mutation of the gsp or GNAS gene, which triggers the adenylyl cyclase system and acts as if GHRH is permissively activated [15]. Alterations in gsp may be seen in about 30–40% of patients with a sporadic GH-secreting tumor. Other alterations include changes in transcription factors (e.g., CREB), cell cycle control genes, both tumor suppressors and oncogenes (e.g., HRas, CCNB2, CCND1, HMGA2, PFGR4, PTTG, Rb, CDKN1B, among many), which are found in 5–15% of tumors, without a clear cut pattern identified to date. Epigenetic alterations (for example, inactivation of CDKN2A (p16), GADD45, and MEG3) have also been identified as having a role in GH adenomagenesis [19].

Younger age of presentation with macroadenomas associated with higher GH levels and poorer responses to medical treatment with somatostatin receptor ligands. The onset of acromegaly in late adolescence or early adulthood is a severe form of acromegaly seen in familial isolated pituitary adenoma [FIPA] associated with aryl hydrocarbon

Disease	Genetic basis	Comments
Multiple endocrine neoplasia Type I	11q13.1	Rare. Autosomal dominant disorder characterized by varying combinations of tumors of parathyroids, pancreatic islets, duodenal endocrine cells, and the anterior pituitary, with 94% penetrance by age 50
Carney complex Type 2	2p16	Rare.. Associated with skin myxomas 62%, cardiac myxomas 30%, Cushing's syndrome 31%, and acromegaly 8% of the patients
McCune-Albright syndrome	20q13.32	Associated with pituitary hyperplasia. Rare. Postzygotic somatic mutation. Classic triad: polyostotic fibrous dysplasia, cafe-au-lait spots with precocious puberty
Familial isolated pituitary adenomas	11q13.2 20q13.32	Rare. Families where 2 cases develop pituitary adenomas
Familial isolated Somatotropinomas	11q13.2 20q13.32	Younger patients. Families where 2 cases of acromegaly with no other endocrine symptoms
PRKAR1A mutations	17q24.2	Rare. Phosphorylation mediated by the cAMP/PKA signaling pathway is involved in the regulation of metabolism, cell proliferation, differentiation, and apoptosis
Aryl hydrocarbon Receptor-interacting Protein	11q13.2	Rare. Ligand-activated transcription factor with resulting complex attains binding specificity for its cognate enhancer elements to regulate transcription of a variety of xenobiotic metabolizing enzymes.
X-linked Acrogigantism	Xq26.3	G-protein coupled receptor 101. Expression of GPR101 cells results in a dose-dependent elevation in reporter activity and intracellular cAMP.

Note: Adapted, in part, from Cuevas-Ramos et al. [18], the Genetics Home Reference (available at: https://ghr.nlm.nih.gov), and the Online Mendelian Inheritance atlas (available at: omim.org).

Table 1.
Genetic mutations and familial acromegaly in GH-secreting pituitary adenoma.

receptor interacting protein alterations [AIP], found on chromosome 11q13 [2]. Somatotroph adenomas are seen in nearly 80% of AIP mutations; in this cohort, the tumors are noted to be more extensive and locally invasive, frequently require re-operation due to rapid or persistent growth despite medical therapy, often require adjuvant radiotherapy; early use of pegvisomant may be needed [20] (see below).

Acromegaly may also present in association with hereditary, autosomal dominant syndromes, multiple endocrine neoplasia type 1 [MEN 1], and Carney Complex [CNC]. MEN1 is caused by a mutation in a tumor suppressor gene located on chromosome 11q13; penetrance is 95% by the age of 55. Roughly 95% of patients have hyperparathyroidism; a pituitary adenoma is seen in 40% or more; and a pancreatic or other foregut tumor is seen in 40% of patients as well. The most common pituitary adenoma is a prolactinoma but somatotropinomas are also seen and may behave more aggressively than sporadic GH-secreting pituitary adenomas; alterations in MEN1 are seen in all MEN1-associated adenomas [21–24]. Mutations in MEN1 can be seen in about 10% of sporadic tumors, similar to the rates noted above [21].

Mild elevations of IGF-1 in the context of pituitary hyperplasia may be seen in patients with genetic syndromes such as the McCune-Albright syndrome and the Carney complex, which clinically may manifest as a subclinical acromegalic syndrome [2]. Lesions may, on rare occasions, grow large enough to cause mass effect and require surgical debulking [25].

4. What is a typical presentation of a patient with acromegaly?

Patients with acromegaly typically present in the fifth decade of life. While 40% of patients are diagnosed by a primary care physician, many are diagnosed because of presentations that lead them to dentists and oral and maxillofacial surgeons, orthopedic, plastic, and podiatric surgeons. or physiatrists and others because of the variegated nature of symptoms and signs, as outlined above [2]. Traditionally, the most common presenting symptoms are orthodontic ones [overbite], enlargement and coarsening of facial features, inability to wear previously well-fitting rings, and increasing shoe size [9]. However, it is also to be noted that a significant minority of patients may not display clear acromegalic features (**Figure 1** and **Table 2**) [27].

5. What comorbidities are commonly associated with acromegaly?

The following co-morbidities are common in patients with acromegaly [2]:

- Cardiovascular disease caused by arterial and left ventricular stiffening, with cardiomyopathy. This is the major cause of mortality in acromegalic patients [28]. Cardiomyopathy excess morbidity and premature mortality can be reduced and in some cases, reversed, by successful treatment [29].

- Hypertension is the most relevant negative prognosticator for mortality in acromegaly and occurs in one-third of all patients [9, 10].

- Abnormal glucose regulation is found in up to a third of acromegalic patients and is an independent prognostic factor of more aggressive disease [10].

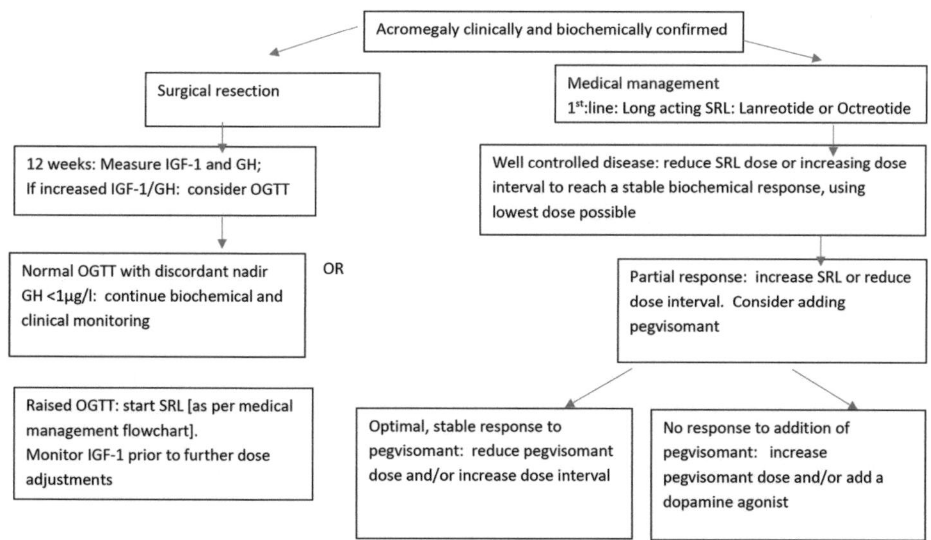

Figure 1.
The acromegaly algorithm. Definitions and notes: SRL: somatostatin receptor ligand, OGTT: oral glucose tolerance test. Algorithm adapted, in part, from Giustina et al. [26] and Capatina and Wass [4].

System	Co-morbidities
Head and neck	• Frontal bossing • Supraorbital ridge bulging • Visual field defects • Enlarged nose, tongue and lips • Prognathism • Mal-occlusion • Tongue hypertrophy +/− sleep apnea
Endocrinological	• Diabetes, glucosuria, abnormal glucose tolerance test • Thyroid gland hypertrophy • Galactorrhea • Menstrual abnormalities • Sexual dysfunction
Cardio-pulmonary	• Cardiomegaly • Systemic Hypertension • Pulmonary Hypertension
Musculoskeletal	• Osteoarthritis • Carpal tunnel syndrome • Enlarged hands • Enlarged feet
Gastro-intestinal	• Hepatomegaly • Nephromegaly • Splenomegaly • Colonic polyps
Miscellaneous	• Skin tags • Hyperhidrosis • Peripheral neuropathy

Table 2.
Anatomical and physiological disturbances associated with acromegaly.

- Vascular morbidity is enhanced by abnormal glucose regulation and hypertension.

- Obstructive sleep apnea caused by swelling of the nasopharyngeal tissue and macroglossia. It may lead to cor pulmonale and right-sided heart failure, which exacerbates the cardiovascular issues outlined above [30]. Musculoskeletal abnormalities: carpal tunnel syndrome and other neurological entrapment syndromes as well as vertebral fractures in presence of normal bone densitometry.

- Thyroid cancer is the most common cancer associated with acromegaly [2].

- Colonic polyps are much more frequent in both incidence and number and require a minimum of one colonoscopy at diagnosis and closer surveillance based on clinical concern. It is controversial whether there is a clear increase in colon cancer in acromegalic patients [26].

- Mass effect: cranial nerve dysfunction, headache, or visual issues due to optic nerve compression (visual field cuts: most commonly, patients present with superior (bi-)temporal hemianopia, before developing loss in the inferior temporal fields; later still, the nasal fields may be involved, but typically not without temporal field defects; visual acuity losses are not common unless the field cuts are extensive) or cranial neuropathy (causing diplopia or ptosis due to involvement of cranial nerves 3, 6, and 4; and rarely causing pain or sensory problems due to involvement of branches of the trigeminal nerve) and pituitary hormonal dysfunction due to a large tumor (macroadenoma) that compresses the normal anterior gland (see **Figure 1**).

6. What is the role of radiological imaging in patients with acromegaly?

The current standard for imaging any pituitary adenoma is magnetic resonance (MR) imaging of the brain with fine cuts (1.5 mm intervals or less) of the brain, without and then with contrast. Field strengths of 1.5tesla or higher are optimal. In some cases, with small or difficult-to-visualize tumors, volumetric, breath-held, fine cut images of the sella may be added.

Over three-fourths of all somatroph adenomas are macroadenomas >1 cm in diameter and are nearly always radiologically detected on MR imaging [31]. In the rare setting in which a fine-cut, high-field sellar MR fails to show an adenoma, a search for an ectopic source of GHRH may need to be done, which is beyond the scope of this review [17].

Somatotroph adenomas, on average, are smaller than most non-functioning or non-secretory macroadenomas; frequently, the tumor will extend into the infrasellar region and involve the sphenoid sinus and clivus [32]. This has been hypothesized based on GH secretion from the presence of normal somatotrophs that tend to be distributed preferentially inferiorly and laterally in the normal pituitary gland, along with the thickening of the diaphragma sella in response to higher GH levels.

7. How is acromegaly diagnosed?

As noted above, neither phenotypic features nor radiological findings comprise distinct, fail-safe diagnostic criteria for acromegaly.

For patients with a suspected pituitary adenoma, biochemical testing is the crux of diagnosis. To evaluate for clinical or sub-clinical acromegaly, one typically measures both GH and IGF-1. The stable plasma levels of IGF-1 correlate with the release of pulsatile GH over 24 h in a log-linear fashion [2]. This pulsatile nature of GH means that isolated, static measures of GH alone cannot be used definitively to make or exclude a diagnosis of acromegaly, since even in the setting of acromegaly, GH secretion remains pulsatile and patients with active disease may have nadir GH levels below the upper limit of normal, just as some normal patients may peak above that limit. Men have random GH levels of <5 ng/mL and women <10 ng/mL as a reference guide in healthy persons. However, as stated above the single, static measure, the IGF-1 level, particularly if it is two times (or higher) than the upper limit of normal for age, sex, and that assay, is the screening test of choice.

If both GH and IGF-1 are markedly elevated, this is pathognomonic for acromegaly, and in the presence of clinical suspicion, an oral glucose tolerance test may not be required [33].

If an oral glucose tolerance test is undertaken, failure of GH to suppress is diagnostic for acromegaly. While the mechanism of glucose-induced GH suppression remains incompletely understood [2] in a healthy person after 100 g of glucose ingestion the GH suppresses to <0–2 ng/mL or undetectable. The high GH nadir value post-oral glucose tolerance test remains the gold standard in the diagnosis of acromegaly.

8. What is the significance of biochemical discordance between GH and IGF-1?

Biochemical discordance between GH and IGF-1 levels is seen in up to one-third of patients with acromegaly; in most patients, the discordance is that of a normal GH and an elevated IGF-1 level. This may be due to polymorphisms of the growth hormone receptor gene [2], which results in increased sensitivity of the receptor to lower GH levels, for example. Additionally, there may be inaccurate laboratory representation of the 24-hour dynamic, pulsatile GH output or technical problems with IGF-1 assays. Growth hormone has a short half-life of 10–20 minutes with IGF-1displaying a longer half-life of hours, of up to a day [7]. Additionally, it has been noted radiotherapy may cause a flat [rather than regular pulsatile] GH secretory pattern [33].

IGF-1, which is synthesized principally in the liver, may be reduced in association with a host of disorders; hepatic failure, renal failure, nutritional [e.g. anorexia], gastrointestinal [e.g. inflammatory bowel disease], endocrine [e.g. hypothyroidism and exogenous estrogens] and metabolic [e.g. type I diabetes mellitus] [2, 33, 34].

9. How is acromegaly monitored?

9.1 Biochemical monitoring of acromegaly

Total IGF-1 levels are noted to reflect GH secretory status accurately. Measurement of free IGF-1 and/or IGF-binding proteins does not provide additional clinical information [33]. The Acromegaly Consensus Group defines 'controlled GH status' biochemically, as optimal disease control, in one of three ways: age and gender-matched IGF-1 levels in the normal range; random GH level of <1.0 micrograms/L; or, a nadir GH, after a properly-conducted OGTT, of <0.4 micrograms/L [34]. Both IGF-1 and GH levels correlate proportionally with mortality, with normalization and decrease of IGF-1 and GH resulting in the mortality of patients decreasing to comparable rates of the general population [33, 34]. Specifically, a random serum GH of less than 1 micrograms/L has been shown to be an indicator of successful treatment and better survival outcomes [30].

Patients on somatostatin receptor ligand (SRL) therapy require regular serial IGF-1 levels and correlated with random GH measurements, In SRL therapy there is no role or indication for the oral glucose tolerance test [33]. Of note, patients on GH receptor antagonist therapy only require serial IGF-1 measurements.

9.2 Comorbidity monitoring

The primary endpoint in the treatment of acromegalic complications is biochemical normalization, which correlates directly with the lowering of the associated

Acromegalic complications	Evaluation and diagnostic tests
• Glucose metabolism • Diabetes acromegalic patients	• Oral glucose tolerance test • Fasting glucose • HbA1C • C peptide
Cardiovascular system	• EKG • Holter EKG monitoring • Echocardiogram • Carotid duplex • BP measurement
Respiratory system	• Polysomnography • Epworth sleep score • Chest CT/MR
Gastrointestinal	• Colonoscopy
Musculoskeletal	• Clinical evaluation • X ray and arthroscopy evaluations

Table 3.
Screening of complications of acromegaly.

morbidities [35]. Over the course of treatment and resultant normalization of serum GH and IGF-1, many comorbidities are attenuated – especially cardiovascular disease, hypertension, and diabetes mellitus - and become comparable to that of the general population [17]. Changes related to bone alterations or joint arthropathies are more resistant to change, such that overall quality of life with successful treatment can be difficult to predict. In general, the longer the duration of untreated or incompletely treated disease, the lower the reduction in or amelioration of acromegalic signs and symptoms (**Table 3**).

10. Do acromegalic patients have a higher morbidity and mortality rate than control populations?

If untreated, acromegaly results in significant, excess morbidity and both acromegaly-related and all-cause mortality when compared to control populations, with standardized mortality ratios of 1.5–2.0 [36]. It is disputed in the literature whether patients with acromegaly have an increase in mortality proportionally to higher GH and IGF-1 levels, although the fractional remission rate can be influential [37].

The increase in the mortality of acromegalic patients is multifactorial. First, there is typically a delay in the diagnosis of acromegaly, with an average interval of 5.2 years [2]. This can result in what may be described as a temporal clustering of patients found in a more advanced state of disease, wherein it is harder, or takes longer, to reverse deleterious pathophysiological effects. Second, the mortality in acromegalic patients is primarily due to cardiovascular and pulmonary effects, which may take longer, to reverse [2].

Other causes of the higher mortality may include cranial radiotherapy, which can lead to accelerated cerebrovascular disease in some; and, more frequently, in between 25 and 50% of patients (depending upon the duration of follow-up and the sensitivity of the pituitary hormone assays that are done) iatrogenic hypopituitarism, which is also known to increase morbidity and mortality, even in the face of appropriate replacement [38, 39].

In 2012, the Safety and Appropriateness of Growth Hormone Treatments in Europe [SAGhE] study evaluated the health of nearly 30,000 patients who had been treated with recombinant growth hormone as children in 1980s. Use of GH was proportionally related to increased bone-tumor mortality [osteosarcoma] and a 7-fold increase in mortality secondary to cerebrovascular disease. There was no evidence of increased risk of colon cancer nor an increase in all-type cancer-related mortality [40].

11. Are there treatment algorithms for acromegaly?

In their most recent report, from 2014, the Acromegaly Consensus Group [26] suggested the following treatment options [4, 33]:

- As noted above, the goal of therapy is to achieve biochemical remission and to maintain it, while minimizing the risk of inducing defects in other pituitary hormones or other conditions.

- In surgically-accessible tumors, or those with mass effects causing neurological compromise, trans-sphenoidal surgery is the treatment of choice.

- Medical treatment with somatotropin analogs in surgically-inaccessible somatotroph adenomas without neurological compromise is reasonable. In some cases, pre-surgical treatment in patients with significant soft tissue swelling or potential airway issues somatostatin analogs have been used, although there is no Level I evidence to support their use. In patients in whom residual disease persists after surgery, or there is recurrent disease that is not resectable, medical therapy is warranted to help normal IGF-1 levels.

- The GH receptor antagonist pegvisomant is considered a treatment option if hormone normalization cannot be not achieved with the other therapies noted above.

- Stereotactic radiosurgery can be a useful, adjuvant treatment option, with two long-term and complementary goals: reduction and control of mass effect and lowering or elimination of GH hypersecretion.

12. What options are available for medical treatment?

Medication may be used as the sole first-line therapeutic option, as an adjuvant to surgical resection in selected cases, or after stereotactic radiosurgery or fractionated radiotherapy to reduce GH levels, after which there is an expected delay in GH levels, one that typically takes 2–5 years for radiosurgery and 3–10 years for fractionated radiation [41]. Periodically after radiation (at 6 or 12-month intervals), one may need to withhold medical therapy for several weeks (for short-acting agents) or longer (for longer-acting agents), to determine whether the radiation has been effective, and this appears to be clinically reasonable, with no rebound hormone levels or increase in tumor size [42].

One must recognize that all treatments for acromegaly, however effective, need to be conceived as having helped the patient achieve remission - and that life-long, clinical and biochemical surveillance is required. In this light, the medical treatment of acromegaly is life-long, thereby liable to cumulative side effects, and with varying efficacy with respect to tumor burden and resistance.

12.1 Somatostatin receptor ligands (Octreotide, Lanreotide and Pasireotide)

Somatostatin receptor ligands [SRLs] are the mainstay and first line of medical treatment of acromegaly. The first generation of SRLs, octreotide and lanreotide, target the somatostatin receptor subtype 2 [2]. Somatostatin subtypes 1,2,4,5 are expressed in both arterial and cardiac myocytes: use of SRLs may reduce the cardiovascular co-morbidities, both by effects on GH excess and, to some degree, by improving diastolic function and ejection fraction, with increased exercise capacity [43]. The variable tumor response rate and corresponding reduction in tumor volume is dependent not only on the physiology of somatostatin receptors, but also on E-cadherin, filamin, and β-arrestin expression (**Tables 4** and 5) [46].

As noted above, SRLs are often used after subtotal resection of a somatotroph adenoma (persistent or recurrent disease) and in the latency period while one awaits radiation therapy to reach full effect [1]. Typically, one maintains the patient on the same dose of SRL for 3 months to adequately assess treatment and determine the need to titrate dosing.

Octreotide comes in two forms, a short-acting form, given three times daily, and a long-acting depot. Long-acting octreotide is administered intramuscularly every 4 weeks and normalizes GH and IGF-1 in up to 79% and 68% of patients respectively; roughly 30–40% of patients will see tumor size reductions that are roughly 30–40% of tumor volume [1]. Lanreotide is available as a depot injection, given every 28 days. It is unclear whether there are significant differences in efficacy rates between octreotide and lanreotide concerning achieving biochemical remission [1]. The maximal benefit of SRL therapy may be achieved in the decade after commencement

Acromegaly-associated comorbidity	Incidence, rate per 10,000 persons-years
Arthropathy/synovitis	4.503
Hypertension	3.908
Hypopituitarism	2.267
Osteoarthritis	2.062
Impaired glucose tolerance test and Diabetes	1.931
Colon polyps	1.554
Cardiac dysrhythmias	1.357
Valvular heart disease	1.343
Sleep apnea	1.301
Menstrual abnormality	1.097
Visual field defects	0.644

Adapted, in part, from Burton et al. [44]. All incidence rates are based on rate per 10,000 person-years.

Table 4.
The incidence of co-morbidities associated with acromegaly.

Medication	Mechanism of action	Goals of treatment	Comments and FDA.gov guidelines
• Octreotide acetate • Sandostatin®	• SSTR2 RL • Long acting octapeptide mimicking somatostatin	To reduce GH and IGF-1 to normal	Begin therapy subcutaneously in an initial dose of 50 mcg three times daily which may be titrated. GH may reduce to normal range in 50% patients IGF-1 reduced to normal in 50–60% of patients
• Lanreotide acetate • Somtuline® depot	• SSTR2 RL • Synthetic analog of somatostatin	To reduce GH and IGF-1 to normal	Dose range is 60–120 mg every 4 weeks. Recommended starting dose is 90 mg deep subcutaneous route every 4 weeks for 3 months, adjustment based on GH and IGF-1 levels. After a single injection of Lanreotide, plasma GH levels fall rapidly and are maintained for at least 28 days
• Pasireotide diaspartate • Signifor®	• SSTR5 > SSTR2 > SSTR3 > SSTR1 multireceptor SRL • Synthetic analog of somatostatin • Binding with high affinity to four of the five SSTRs	To reduce GH and IGF-1 to normal	Indicated in patients with an inadequate response to surgery and/or for whom surgery is not an option. Recommended initial dosage is either 0.6 mg or 0.9 mg by subcutaneous route twice a day. Titrate dosage in response to treatment [reduction in 24-h urinary free cortisol] and symptomatology.
Cabergoline dostinex®	Long acting dopamine receptor agonist with high affinity for D2 receptors	To normalize IGF-I levels Consider for cdenoma co-secreting PRL and GH [45]	Cardiovascular examination prior to therapy commencement to rule out valvulopathy. Recommended dosage for initiation of therapy is 1.0 mg orally once or twice a week with adjustment until normalization of IGF-1 levels.
Bromocriptine Parlodel®	Ergot derivative with potent dopamine receptor agonist activity	To reduce GH levels Consider for cdenoma co-secreting PRL and GH	Initial recommended oral dosage is 1.25 mg to 2.5 mg daily, with increments of 2.5 mg biweekly until therapeutic response. Alone or as adjunctive therapy with pituitary irradiation or surgery, reduces serum growth hormone by 50% or more in approximately half of acromegalic patients treated, although not usually to normal levels
• Pegvisomant • Somavert®	• GH-receptor antagonist • Analog of human growth hormone (GH) that has been structurally altered to act as a GH receptor antagonist	To normalize IGF-I levels	Recommended loading dose of 40 mg given subcutaneously with increase every 4–6 weeks Indicated in patients with an inadequate response to surgery and/or as a second-line treatment in whom the above therapies are contraindicated.

SSTR Somatostatin Receptors, IGF-1 insulin-like growth factor, GH growth hormone PRL prolactin.

Table 5.
Medical therapy used in acromegaly.

in approximately 70% of patients. SRL therapy is generally well tolerated, with 1 in 10 patients describing transient gastrointestinal symptoms (like diarrhea, abdominal discomfort, nausea, and flatulence) due to the inhibition of pancreatic exocrine secretions [47]. In rare cases (less than 1 in 100 patients), side effects may include glucose intolerance, steatorrhea requiring the introduction of pancreatic enzymes, and hair loss due to thyroid issues [48]. A meta-analysis showed first-generation SRLs to statistically decrease fasting serum insulin, with minor overall clinical impact on acromegaly, irrespective of the use of octreotide or lanreotide [49]. Medical treatment pre-operatively with SRL, as discussed above, has not been demonstrated, in any controlled, randomized, and blinded studies, to improve surgical outcomes or reduce any post-operative complications [8].

The options for patients with resistance to first-generation SRLs include, but are not limited to: higher dosing, combination with pegvisomant and/or cabergoline, and, more recently, the use of pasireotide [46]. Pasireotide is a next-generation SRL with broader somatostatin receptor patterns of interaction with 4 of the 5 SST receptors, particularly somatostatin receptor 5. Pasireotide is given as an intramuscular injection, every 4 weeks. The side effect profile of intramuscular pasireotide is similar to that of first-generation agents, however, a for a higher incidence of hyperglycemia-related adverse events with pasireotide, requiring closer monitoring of the patient's glycemic status [50].

12.2 Growth hormone receptor antagonist (Pegvisomant)

Pegvisomant is a mutated analog of human growth hormone, with highly selective ligand affinity for growth hormone receptor binding sites 2 and 5. When it binds to the GH receptor, it prevents functionally correct receptor dimerization [51]. Pegvisomant is administered subcutaneously once daily.

The ACROSTUDY showed pegvisomant to be an effective, single medical treatment option for patients with acromegaly, with approximately two-thirds (65.8%) of subjects achieving and maintaining IGF-1 normalization at 5-year follow-up [43, 52]. Serum IGF-1 concentrations show a dose-dependent decrease, with 75% of the final maximal reduction occurring within the first 2 weeks of administration [51]. As would be expected in an agent that lowers IGF-1 by blocking the GH receptor, many patients will have a compensatory rise in the GH level. The most common side effects include liver enzyme abnormalities in 2.5% of patients, administration site reactions in the form of lipodystrophy in 2.3%, and a comparable rate of tumor growth in 10 of 710 patients who were on pegvisomant alone [49].

In general, pegvisomant is reserved for patients with persistently elevated IGF-1 levels despite maximizing other treatment modalities [1, 2]. It may also be used in conjunction with an SRL, or even cabergoline or bromocriptine, especially in patients that have elevated levels of GH and prolactin (mixed somatomammotropinomas) [8]. Pegvisomant is significantly more expensive than most SLRs. Given the expense, it has been suggested that at least a 2/3rds reduction in actual cost would make pegvisomant more cost effective relative to the other medical agents, certainly to become a widely used first line medication [9].

12.3 DAs: dopamine agonist (cabergoline)

Dopamine agonists, such as cabergoline or bromocriptine, decrease GH (and prolactin) secretion. Typically, they are used as complementary, adjuvant therapy with SRLs, since monotherapy with DA is effective in roughly 10% of patients or fewer [8]. Oral dopamine agonists, as noted above, may be useful in patients whose tumors secrete both prolactin and GH [43].

DAs are generally not used in patients with Parkinson's Disease patients. An association between long-term, high-dose therapy and clinically relevant cardiac valvular disease remains controversial and uncertain [8].

13. What are the surgical options in acromegaly?

Surgical resection is the first-line, gold standard, and the most efficacious treatment option for patients with microadenomas and macroadenomas without extracellular invasion [1, 9, 42, 53]. Both the microsurgical transsphenoidal and endonasal, endoscopic transsphenoidal routes are utilized to access pituitary adenomas. Surgical resection results in both a rapid reduction of the tumor mass effect on surrounding structures (cranial nerve palsies and optic chiasm) and a reduction in hormonal secreting tumor bulk, with normalization of IGF-1 levels in 6–12 weeks after total resection (recognizing the half-life of IGF-1).

After surgery, biochemical normalization is seen in 50–95% of patients. Tumor volume and invasion of parasellar structures (bone, dura, or cavernous sinus walls or contents) as the best predictors of both the limits of resection and of hormone normalization [54]. Thus, hormone control rates are lower in patients with macroadenomas when compared to those with microadenomas; and patients in whom the bone, dura, or cavernous sinus are invaded, have continued reductions in surgical remission rates associated with lower control rates [42]. Even with large and invasive tumors, remission rates in patients where trans-sphenoidal surgery is combined, deliberately, with adjunctive multimodal therapy, long-term remission rates can exceed 80% [55].

In cases with residual disease, medication [usually SRLs] or postoperative radiation therapy is recommended [56]. The complication rate for transsphenoidal surgery is surgeon experience dependent, usually quoted as less than 5% and this includes infection (sinusitis; less commonly, meningitis), hyponatremia, CSF leak, anterior pituitary hormone deficiencies, diabetes insipidus, cranial neuropathies, and vision perturbations.

Cranial approaches are rarely needed and are generally reserved for patients with large tumors that invade the intracranial spaces and cause neurological compromise. The craniotomy is done to achieve maximal, safe resection as part of a multi-modality approach that will likely also include medication and radiation to achieve long-term mass and hormone control.

14. What is the role of radiation therapy in acromegaly?

Conventional radiotherapy is delivered as single beams of high-energy radiation in fractionated, daily doses given over 5–6 weeks, typically for a cumulative dose in the range of 50 Gy [53, 57]. The risk of adverse effects is proportional to the daily fractionated dose and the maximal dose. At present, most centers use conformal techniques of intensity-modulated radiation therapy [IMRT] to reduce the radiation dose to normal intracranial structures. IMRT may be considered a safe alternative option for residual or recurrent tumors close to the optic chiasm [within 2 mm] [42].

The pre-radiotherapy levels of GH and IGF-1 are the most important factors in the eventual success of radiation therapy in acromegaly [30]. In patients undergoing

IMRT, the higher the pre-treatment GH and IGF-1 levels (off medication), the longer it takes to achieve remission and the lower the overall success remission rate with radiation alone [57]. Although the greatest reduction in GH levels after IMRT is in the first 24–36 months, it may take a decade or longer to achieve biochemical remission and normalization of IGF-1 levels [57]. As one may conceive, this long latency period means that radiation is not a first-line treatment option for patients with acromegaly, for the reasons discussed above. Depending upon how long (years versus decades) and how extensively one screens patients for hypopituitarism after radiation, anterior hormone deficiency ranges from 25% to as high as 80% in some studies [1, 35, 51, 57]. Other delayed deficits of radiation therapy include visual deficits (approximately 5%), radiation necrosis (on the order of 1%), and an increase in cerebrovascular disease since the large cerebral vessels at the base of the skull are included in the field [57].

15. What is the role of stereotactic radiosurgery (SRS) in acromegaly?

Stereotactic radiosurgery (SRS) has emerged as a useful, adjuvant treatment modality option for well-selected patients with residual tumors after surgery and some on medical treatment. Typically, to be a candidate, the tumor needs to be at least 2 mm from the optic nerve, chiasm, or radiation; this may be the lower limit for frame-based methods – it may be greater than 2 mm when treating with frameless techniques, since the former may have slightly better accuracy, because the head is fixed rigidly during treatment [1, 42, 53]. SRS consists of multiple, low-energy beams forming a dosimetric map around the target, with a suprathreshold integral dose, but sharp radioactivity falls off beyond the target [57]. There are several brands of SRS that differ in the method used, including Gamma Knife® (Elekta, Stockholm, Sweden), which uses a cobalt-60 source to generate gamma rays; Cyberknife® (Accuray, Sunnyvale, CA), a linear particle accelerator that generates 6MV x-ray irradiation); or proton-beam radiosurgery.

SRS is usually administered as an outpatient, one-day, single-dose treatment. Over the long-term of 3–5 years, SRS may be more cost-effective than the life-long medical treatment options of SRLs and GHRAs [1]. The mean radiation dose to the margin of the pituitary adenoma in most patients is 16-20Gy, striving to at least achieve 15Gy to the equivalent of the 50% local isodose line (the outer aspect of the tumor, with doses increasing inside the mass of the tumor to essentially twice the 50% isodose) [57, 58]. One strives to minimize the dose to normal, para sellar structures, especially the optic apparatus, trying to keep the dose to 9Gy or less, if possible [53]. IMRT and SRS have comparable incidences of hormone normalization and hypopituitarism, although SRS tends to effect biochemical remission faster, typically in 2–5 years in 70–80% of those patients treated with SRS, compared to 3–10 years for IMRT [42, 53].

There are several key points to consider:

- The greater the maximal radiation dose (that can be delivered safely) significantly predicts hormonal remission. Interestingly, the marginal radiation dose is not prognostically significant [53].
- The radiation dose to the pituitary stalk directly correlates to the degree of hypopituitarism [42].
- Mass control means the tumor stays the same size as well as, in many patients, becoming smaller. However, not all tumors get smaller, even if the tumor cells no

longer secrete or die. It is therefore important to recognize that in some patients, hormone normalization is not directly associated with a reduction in the tumor size post-radiation. In this setting, neuroimaging may be misleading; biochemical monitoring of IGF-1 is the crux of long-term follow-up [35, 57].

- Some small, non-controlled, retrospective studies in which somatostatin analogs were given at the time of radiation, suggested that concurrent use may decrease the efficacy of radiation by decreasing the proliferation rate of the adenoma, as indicated by lower GH levels [35, 53]. Some advocate holding off on medical therapy for 1–2 months and 1–3 months after radiation, to take advantage of any DNA damage that radiation may cause to proliferating tumor cells. This remains an unclear area.

- Compared to radiation therapy, SRS has a shorter mean remission time, of 3.3 years, with late-onset hypopituitarism (more than 5 years later), which may affect up to 50% of patients [1, 42]. The second most common adverse effect is optic neuropathy, which occurs in fewer than 1% of patients [57].

16. Conclusion

This paper reviews the current management options for the management of acromegaly, including the various options of medical treatment, radiation therapy, and surgical options.

Learning objectives

Identify the clinical and biochemical features of acromegaly.

Discuss the treatment options for patients with acromegaly to compare and understand the risks and rationale of each treatment strategy.

Understand the accompanying comorbidities of acromegaly requiring long-term surveillance and treatment.

Key points

In approximately 95% of patients, acromegaly is caused by a somatotroph adenoma, with excess secretion of growth hormone after epiphyseal plate closure resulting in symptoms and signs due to hypertrophic changes in bones, muscles, joints, and soft tissues without changes in height. Before epiphyseal plate closure this results in excessive vertical and appendicular growth in children and adolescents.

In <5% of the patient population, acromegaly is secondary to ectopic growth hormone releasing hormone (GHRH) or a growth hormone-secreting neuroendocrine tumor.

- Acromegaly is characterized by chronically elevated growth hormone [GH] and insulin-like growth factor-1 [IGF-1] serum levels.

- On presentation, acromegalic patients may have involvement of multiple systems: cardiovascular, respiratory, metabolic, bones, and joints, resulting in elevated morbidity and premature mortality rates compared to age- and sex-matched patients without acromegaly.

- For most patients, trans-nasal surgical resection of the adenoma is the preferred option, due to its ability to effect rapid and lasting biochemical cure, with long-term (5+ years) remission rates of 80–90% in microadenomas, with decreasing surgical efficacy as tumors increase in size and extent of parasellar invasion of the bone, dura, cavernous and paranasal air sinuses, and intracranial spaces.

- Other therapeutic options for acromegaly include lifelong medical treatments with one or more of a variety of agents, including somatostatin ligand receptors, growth hormone receptor antagonists, and dopamine agonists. For some patients, especially those with invasive tumors and those who have incomplete responses to medical treatment, radiotherapy may be useful. Both stereotactic radiosurgery and fractionated radiation therapy can treat both the mass effect and reduce and, possibly, eliminate the hypersecretory states.

Author details

Maleeha Ahmad[1*] and Robert J. Weil[2]

1 Department of Neurosurgery, Loma Linda University, Loma Linda, CA, United States

2 Southcoast Physicians Group, Dartmouth, MA, United States

*Address all correspondence to: ahmadm.neurosurgeon@gmail.com

References

[1] Marko NF, LaSota E, Hamrahian AH, Weil RJ. Comparative effectiveness review of treatment options for pituitary microadenomas in acromegaly. Journal of Neurosurgery. 2012;**117**(3):522-538

[2] Ribeiro-Oliveira A Jr, Barkan A. The changing face of acromegaly – Advances in diagnosis and treatment. Nature Reviews. Endocrinology. 2012;**8**(10):605-611

[3] Melmed S. Medical progress: Acromegaly. The New England Journal of Medicine. 2006;**355**(24):2558-2573

[4] Capatina C, Wass JA. 60 Years of neuroendocrinology: Acromegaly. The Journal of Endocrinology. 2015;**226**(2):T141-T160

[5] Lin-Su K, Wajnrajch MP. Growth hormone releasing hormone (GHRH) and the GHRH receptor. Reviews in Endocrine & Metabolic Disorders. 2002;**3**(4):313-323

[6] Natelson BH, Holaday J, Meyerhoff J, Stokes PE. Temporal changes in growth hormone, cortisol, and glucose: Relation to light onset and behavior. The American Journal of Physiology. 1975;**229**(2):409

[7] Clemmons DR. Clinical laboratory indices in the treatment of acromegaly. Clinica Chimica Acta. 2011;**412**(5-6):403-409

[8] Melmed S, Colao A, Barkan A, Molitch M, Grossman AB, Kleinberg D, et al. Guidelines for acromegaly management: An update. Journal of Clinical Endocrinology & Metabolism. 2009;**94**(5):1509-1517

[9] Kimmell KT, Weil RJ, Marko NF. Multi-modal management of acromegaly: A value perspective. Pituitary. 2015;**18**(5):658-665

[10] Sherlock M, Ayuk J, Tomlinson JW, Toogood AA, Aragon-Alonso A, Sheppard MC, et al. Mortality in patients with pituitary disease. Endocrine Reviews. 2010;**31**(3):301-342

[11] Asa SL, Eaazt S. The pathogenesis of pituitary tumors. Annual Review of Pathology: Mechanisms of Disease. 2009;**4**:97-126

[12] Orija IB, Weil RJ, Hamrahian AH. Pituitary incidentaloma. Best Practice & Research Clinical Endocrinology & Metabolism. 2012;**26**(1):47

[13] Vernooij MW, Ikram MA, Tanghe HL, Vincent AJ, Hofman A, Krestin GP, et al. Incidental findings on brain MRI in the general population. The New England Journal of Medicine. 2007;**357**(18):1821

[14] Hall WA, Luciano MG, Doppman JL, Patronas NJ, Oldfield EH. Pituitary magnetic resonance imaging in normal human volunteers: Occult adenomas in the general population. Annals of Internal Medicine. 1994;**120**(10):817

[15] Lopes MBS. Growth hormone-secreting adenomas: Pathology and cell biology. Neurosurgical Focus. 2010;**29**(4):E2

[16] Kreutzer J, Vance ML, Lopes MB, Laws ERJ. Surgical management of GH-secreting pituitary adenomas: An outcome study using modern remission criteria. Journal of Clinical Endocrinology & Metabolism. 2001;**86**(9):4072-4077

[17] Daud S, Hamrahian AH, Weil RJ, Hamaty M, Prayson RA, Olansky L.

Acromegaly with negative pituitary MRI and no evidence of ectopic source: The role of transphenoidal pituitary exploration? Pituitary. 2011;**14**(4):414-417

[18] Cuevas-Ramos D, Fleseriu M. Pasireotide: A novel treatment for patients with acromegaly. Dovepress. 2016;**2016**(10):227

[19] Pack SD, Qin LX, Pak E, Wang Y, Ault DO, Mannan P, et al. Common genetic changes in hereditary and sporadic pituitary adenomas detected by comparative genomic hybridization. Genes, Chromosomes & Cancer. 2005;**43**(1):72-82

[20] Daly AF, Tichomirowa MA, PetrossiansP,HeliovaaraE,Jaffrain-ReaML, Barlier A, et al. Clinical characteristics and therapeutic responses in patients with germ-line AIP mutations and pituitary adenomas: An international collaborative study. The Journal of Clinical Endocrinology and Metabolism. 2010;**95**(11):E373-E383

[21] Zhuang Z, Ezzat SZ, Vortmeyer AO, Weil R, Oldfield EH, Park WS, et al. Mutations of the MEN1 tumor suppressor gene in pituitary tumors. Cancer Research. 1997;**57**(24):5446-5451

[22] Weil RJ, Vortmeyer AO, Huang S, Boni R, Lubensky IA, Pack S, et al. 11q13 allelic loss in pituitary tumors in patients with multiple endocrine neoplasia syndrome type 1. Clinical Cancer Research. 1998;**4**(7):1673-1678

[23] Weil RJ, Huang S, Pack S, Vortmeyer AO, Tsokos M, Lubensky IA, et al. Pluripotent tumor cells in benign pituitary adenomas associated with multiple endocrine neoplasia type 1. Cancer Research. 1998;**58**(20):4715-4720

[24] Schernthaner-Reiter MH, Trivellin G, Stratakis CA. MEN1, MEN4, and carney complex: Pathology and molecular genetics. Neuroendocrinology. 2016;**103**(1):18-31. DOI: 10.1159/000371819. Epub 2015 Jan 9. PMID: 25592387; PMCID: PMC4497946

[25] Vortmeyer AO, Gläsker S, Mehta GU, Abu-Asab MS, Smith JH, Zhuang Z, et al. Somatic GNAS mutation causes widespread and diffuse pituitary disease in acromegalic patients with McCune-Albright syndrome. The Journal of Clinical Endocrinology and Metabolism. 2012;**97**(4):2403

[26] Giustina A, Chanson P, Kleinberg D, Bronstein MD, Clemmons DR, Klibanski A, et al. Expert consensus document: A consensus on the medical treatment of acromegaly. Nature Reviews. Endocrinology. 2014;**10**(4):243-248

[27] Wade AN, Baccon J, Grady MS, Judy KD, O'Rourke DM, Snyder PJ. Clinically silent somatotroph adenomas are common. European Journal of Endocrinology. 2011;**165**(1):39-44

[28] Vance ML. Acromegaly: A fascinating pituitary disorder. Introduction. Neurosurgical Focus. 2010;**29**(4):ntrouton

[29] Mosca S, Paolillo S, Colao A, Bossone E, Cittadini A, Iudice FL, et al. Cardiovascular involvement in patients affected by acromegaly: An appraisal. International Journal of Cardiology. 2013;**167**(5):1712

[30] McCabe J, Ayuk J, Sherlock M. Treatment factors that influence mortality in acromegaly. Neuroendocrinology. 2015

[31] Lonser RR, Kindzelski BA, Mehta GU, Jane JA Jr, Oldfield EH. Acromegaly without imaging evidence of pituitary adenoma. The Journal of Clinical Endocrinology and Metabolism. 2010;**95**(9):4192-4196

[32] Zada G, Lin N, Laws ER Jr. Patterns of extrasellar extension in growth hormone-secreting and nonfunctional pituitary macroadenomas. Neurosurgical Focus. 2010;**29**(4):E4

[33] Giustina A, Chanson P, Bronstein MD, Klibanski A, Lamberts S, Casanueva FF, et al. A consensus on criteria for cure of acromegaly. The Journal of Clinical Endocrinology and Metabolism. 2010;**95**(7):3141-3148

[34] Melmed S, Kleinberg DL, Bonert V, Fleseriu M. Acromegaly: Assessing the disorder and navigating therapeutic options for treatment. Endocr Pract. 2014 quiz 18-20; Oct;20(Suppl. 1):7-17.

[35] Castinetti F, Regis J, Dufour H, Brue T. Role of stereotactic radiosurgery in the management of pituitary adenomas. Nature Reviews. Endocrinology. 2010 Apr;**6**(4):214-223

[36] Hazer DB, Isik S, Berker D, Guler S, Gurlek A, Yucel T, et al. Treatment of acromegaly by endoscopic transsphenoidal surgery: Surgical experience in 214 cases and cure rates according to current consensus criteria. Journal of Neurosurgery. 2013 Dec;**119**(6):1467-1477

[37] Colao A, Auriemma RS, Lombardi G, Pivonello R. Resistance to somatostatin analogs in acromegaly. Endocrine Reviews. 2011 Apr;**32**(2):247-271

[38] Lindholm J, Nielsen EH, Bjerre P, Christiansen JS, Hagen C, Juul S, et al. Hypopituitarism and mortality in pituitary adenoma. Clinical Endocrinology. 2006;**65**(1):51

[39] Pappachan JM, Raskauskiene D, Kutty VR, Clayton RN. Excess mortality associated with hypopituitarism in adults: A meta-analysis of observational studies. The Journal of Clinical Endocrinology and Metabolism. 2015;**100**(4):1405

[40] Carel J, Ecosse E, Landier F, Meguellati-Hakkas D, Kaguelidou F, Rey G, et al. Long-term mortality after recombinant growth hormone treatment for isolated growth hormone deficiency or childhood short stature: Preliminary report of the French SAGhE study. Journal of Clinical Endocrinology & Metabolism. 2012 Feb;**97**(2):416-425

[41] Abu Dabrh A, Asi N, Farah W, Mohammed K, Wang Z, Farah M, et al. Radiotherapy vs. radiosurgery in treating patients with acromegaly: Systematic review and meta-analysis. Endocrine Practice. 18 Mar 2015:1-33. DOI: 10.4158/EP14574.RA. PMID: 25786558 [Epub ahead of print]

[42] Oldfield EH. Editorial: Unresolved issues: Radiosurgery versus radiation therapy; medical suppression of growth hormone production during radiosurgery; and endoscopic surgery versus microscopic surgery. Neurosurgical Focus. 2010;**29**(4):E16

[43] Colao A. Improvement of cardiac parameters in patients with acromegaly treated with medical therapies. Pituitary. 2012;**15**(1):50-58

[44] Burton T, Le Nestour E, Bancroft T, Neary M. Real-world comorbidities and treatment patterns of patients with acromegaly in two large US health plan databases. Pituitary. 2013;**16**(3):354-362

[45] Abs R, Verhelst J, Maiter D, Van Acker K, Nobels F, Coolens JL, et al. Cabergoline in the treatment of acromegaly: A study in 64 patients. The Journal of Clinical Endocrinology and Metabolism. 1998;**83**(2):374

[46] Gadelha MR, Wildemberg LE, Bronstein MD, Gatto F, Ferone D. Somatostatin receptor ligands in the

treatment of acromegaly. Pituitary. 2017;**20**(1):100

[47] Gariani K, Meyer P, Philippe J. Implications of somatostatin analogs in the treatment of acromegaly. US Endocrinology. 2013;**9**(1):62

[48] Edling KLHA. An update on the treatment of acromegaly. Research and Reports in Endocrine Disorders. 2013;**3**:1

[49] Mazziotti G, Floriani I, Bonadonna S, Torri V, Chanson P, Giustina A. Effects of somatostatin analogs on glucose homeostasis: A metaanalysis of acromegaly studies. The Journal of Clinical Endocrinology and Metabolism. 2009;**94**(5):1500

[50] McKeage K. Pasireotide in acromegaly: A review. Drugs. 2015;**75**(9):1039-1048

[51] Trainer PJ, Drake WM, Katznelson L, Freda PU, Herman-Bonert V, van der Lely AJ, et al. Treatment of acromegaly with the growth hormone-receptor antagonist pegvisomant. The New England Journal of Medicine. 2000;**342**(16):1171-1177

[52] Freda PU, Gordon MB, Kelepouris N, Jonsson P, Koltowska-Haggstrom M, van der Lely AJ. Long-term treatment with pegvisomant as monotherapy in patients with acromegaly: Experience from acrostudy. Endocrine Practice. 2015;**21**(3):264-274

[53] Stapleton CJ, Liu CY, Weiss MH. The role of stereotactic radiosurgery in the multimodal management of growth hormone-secreting pituitary adenomas. Neurosurgical Focus. 2010;**29**(4):E11

[54] Hofstetter CP, Mannaa RH, Mubita L, Anand VK, Kennedy JW, Dehdashti AR, et al. Endoscopic endonasal transsphenoidal surgery for growth hormone-secreting pituitary adenomas. Neurosurgical Focus. 2010;**29**(4):E6

[55] Swearingen B, Barker FG 2nd, Katznelson L, Biller BM, Grinspoon S, Klibanski A, et al. Long-term mortality after transsphenoidal surgery and adjunctive therapy for acromegaly. The Journal of Clinical Endocrinology and Metabolism. 1998;**83**(10):3419-3426

[56] Gondim JA, Almeida JP, de Albuquerque LAF, Gomes E, Schops M, Ferraz T. Pure endoscopic transsphenoidal surgery for treatment of acromegaly: Results of 67 cases treated in a pituitary center. Neurosurgical Focus. 2010;**29**(4):E7

[57] Rowland NC, Aghi MK. Radiation treatment strategies for acromegaly. Neurosurgical Focus. 2010;**29**(4):E12

[58] Muh CR, Oyesiku NM. Pituitary tumors. In: Ellenbogen R, editor. Principles of Neurological Surgery. Third ed. 2012. pp. 621-644

Chapter 2

Using a Precision Approach to Optimize the Drug Therapy of Patients with Acromegaly Syndrome

Vyacheslav S. Pronin, Mikhail B. Antsiferov, Tatyana M. Alekseeva and Evgeny V. Pronin

Abstract

Modern problems of acromegaly treatment are associated with the heterogeneous composition of somatotrophic tumors, differing in clinical course and sensitivity to the proposed therapy. Under these conditions, the achievement of acromegaly control depends on the stratification of clinical, laboratory and instrumental data in order to identify significant biomarkers that allow predicting the receptor phenotype and biological behavior of the tumor, the tendency to relapse and the long-term effectiveness of drug therapy. The review discusses modern predictor models reflecting the radicality of surgical treatment, the risk of the continued growth of a resident tumor, the long-term results of clinical use of first-generation somatostatin receptor ligands (fg-SRLs), as well as the possibilities of therapeutic maneuver. It is proposed to use pharmacotherapeutic testing to evaluate the receptor expression of tumor cells and predict the effectiveness of long-term treatment of fg-SRLs. Summary data characterizing various morphotypes of somatotrophic tumors are presented. It is shown that the use of a precision approach can significantly accelerate the time to achieve control and improve the quality of the treatment aid in patients with acromegaly syndrome.

Keywords: acromegaly syndrome, somatotrophic tumors, prognostic factors, drug therapy, somatostatin analogs

1. Introduction

Acromegaly is an insidious chronic disease with a great burden resulting from: insufficient medical awareness, delayed diagnosis and undifferentiated formal therapy. The cumulative effect of excessive secretion of growth hormone (GH) and insulin-like growth factor – 1 (IGF-1) contributes to the formation of specific somatic, systemic and metabolic disorders in the body, often of an irreversible nature. In the absence of adequate treatment, the disease is characterized by high rates of morbidity and premature mortality associated with the development of cardiovascular, respiratory, metabolic and neoplastic disorders. A direct correlation between the duration of uncontrolled disease and the severity of combined life-threatening complications has been proven. Independent predictors of premature death include: cardiovascular disorders; arterial hypertension; diabetes mellitus; high levels of GH and IGF-I persisting, despite ongoing treatment; long duration of the active stage; elderly age of patients [1–3].

According to epidemiological data, the prevalence of acromegaly in terms of circulation is 28–137 cases and the incidence is 2–11 cases per 1 million inhabitants [4]. An important problem is the delayed diagnosis of acromegaly, which is associated with the slow course of the disease, insufficient awareness of this pathology among practitioners, as well as a low level of dispensary supervision. It is shown that in 54% of patients, the prediagnostic period is more than 10 years, which contributes to the development of irreversible multiple organ complications and negatively affects the quality and life expectancy of patients. At the time of detection, most of the tumors are macroadenomas possibly relating to diagnostic delays and posing challenges in surgical management. Currently, the direction of early diagnosis of the disease is actively developing, including various methods of mass and selective screening, proving that the actual prevalence of acromegaly significantly exceeds the existing indicators for the treatment [5–7].

2. Acromegaly syndrome

Contrary to previous ideas, acromegaly is not a monomorphic disease but is a syndrome that unites a group of morphologically and functionally different formations. In the 5th Edition of the 2022 WHO Classification of Head and Neck Neuroendocrine Neoplasms, pituitary somatotrophic adenomas are referred to as somatotrophic pituitary neuroendocrine tumors (PitNET). There are at least six distinct genetically determined or sporadic morphologic types PitNET, which, despite belonging to a single PIT1-dependent family and a common acidophilic cell line, nevertheless differ in histological structure, hormonal and proliferative activity, aggressiveness of intracranial growth and sensitivity to the treatment presented [8, 9].

From differentiated histological subtypes, pure—Densely Granulated and Sparsely Granulated Somatotroph Tumors, Mammosomatotroph Tumors and mixed—somatotroph–lactotroph tumors are distinguished. Low-differentiated morphotypes (Mature Plurihormonal Tumors of PIT1-Lineage, Immature PIT1-Lineage Tumors, Acidophil Stem Cell Tumors), characterized by low secretory activity but accelerated invasive growth are also described [10, 11].

The most common variant, occurring in 30–50% of cases, are sporadic Densely Granulated Somatotroph Tumors (DGST), formed during 4–6 decades of life and characterized by preserved species specialization, slow growth and high secretory activity. In addition to GH, DGST secretes an α-subunit (α-SU), the determination of which may have differential diagnostic value. This form of acromegaly is characterized by late manifestation, latent nature of the course and poorly expressed orofacial changes, which is manifested, as a rule, by delayed diagnosis and a wide range of disabling multiple organ and metabolic disorders that negatively affect the quality and life expectancy of patients. Nevertheless, the preservation of the receptor phenotype with the dominant expression of the 2nd subtype of somatostatin receptors (SSTR2) in DGST cells is manifested by good sensitivity to first-generation somatostatin receptor ligands (fg-SRLs) [12, 13].

In 15–35% of cases, the cause of acromegaly is less differentiated Sparsely Granulated Somatotroph Tumors (SGST), manifested by accelerated extracellular and invasive growth, leading to the development of intracranial compression, visual and neurovascular disorders. These tumors are typically invasive macrotumors with extrasellar invasion at the time of diagnosis. In SGST cells, there is a relatively lower density of SSTR2, which causes resistance to fg-SRLs. Increased proliferative index Ki-67 (>3%) and low content of the adhesive protein E-cadherin contribute to the active and invasive character of tumor growth. This subtype of somatotrophic adenomas, which is the most problematic for curation, manifests at a young age and is characterized by a pronounced mass effect, a reviving course and resistance to radiation and drug effects. Due to the high risk of malignancy, SGST is included in the group of aggressive neuroendocrine pituitary tumors requiring active combined treatment and lifelong dynamic control [10, 14].

The biological behavior of mixed somato-lactotrophic tumors and their sensitivity to treatment are determined by the cytological composition of the somatotrophic component of a bicellular tumor and, in the presence of rarely granular cells, these tumors also differ in a negative therapeutic prognosis. Mammosomatotrophic tumors belong to monocellular adenomas, in which each cell secretes GH and prolactin, and are characterized by hereditary predisposition, early manifestation (active linear growth) and high secretory activity. Since these tumors consist of densely granular cells, they differ in sensitivity to fg-SRLs and low signal intensity on T2-weighted MR images. In addition, rare PIT1-line tumors (plurihormonal and poorly differentiated neoplasms, as well as acidophilic stem cell tumors) are isolated, which are characterized by invasive growth and a negative prognosis.

Most of the GH-secreting tumors are sporadic. In 40% of cases, a somatic mutation of the gene encoding the synthesis of the alpha subunit of the receptor G protein *(GNAS1)* is observed, contributing to an increase in the secretory and mitogenic activity of cells. Approximately 4–12% of patients have a congenital mutation of the gene responsible for the synthesis of aryl hydrocarbon receptor-interacting protein *(AIP)*. This form occurs in young patients and is manifested by accelerated and invasive growth of the pituitary tumor. In about 5% of cases, clinical symptom complexes are observed due to congenital genetic disorders (MEN syndromes of types 1 and 4, Carney complex, McCune-Albright syndrome, familial isolated pituitary adenoma, X-linked acrogiantism, etc.). These tumors manifest at an early age, are clinically manifested by gigantism, and are characterized by rapid growth, aggressive course and resistance to treatment. The extrahypophysial causes of acromegaly, detected in 1% of cases, include ectopic neuroendocrine tumors secreting GH or somatoliberin, the visualization and treatment of which are often a clinical problem [13–15].

3. Tumor-oriented diagnosis and treatment

Thus, the existing intra-group differences in the biological behavior of GH-secreting adenomas, their ability to residual growth, and susceptibility to drugs dictate the need for a tumor-oriented differential diagnostic search to establish a specific immunohistochemical subtype of a somatotrophic tumor as an indispensable condition for the development of an effective therapeutic aid. Unfortunately, the neglect of the syndrome approach observed in clinical practice manifests itself in the unified pharmacotherapy schemes of the acromegaly method “a trial-and-error” with the “blind” selection of a suitable drug, which, in case of an incorrect decision, is fraught with further progression of the disease and shortening of the survival period. The precision approach in endocrinological practice involves the use of clinical, humoral, imaging and pathomorphological predictors for preliminary stratification of clinically homogeneous patients with a clear clinical prognosis and response to treatment [16, 17].

Currently, individual biomarkers capable of predicting the possibility of postoperative remission, the risk of recurrence (or continued growth of a residual tumor), as well as the long-term effectiveness of drug therapy (DT), taking into account the immunological phenotype and clinical characteristics of PitNET, are widely discussed in the scientific literature. For example, it has been established that the intensity of the tumor signal on T2-weighted magnetic imaging can indirectly indicate the morphological variant of somatotrophic tumors and, accordingly, predict sensitivity to SRL treatment. Thus, DGST is manifested by a low signal intensity compared to surrounding formations (the intact part of the pituitary gland, gray or white matter of the cerebral cortex), whereas SGST is characterized by a high signal intensity. The introduction of this diagnostic feature into domestic clinical practice will make it easier to choose a treatment strategy [18–20].

It is proved that persistent biochemical control is the main factor determining the quality of life and survival of patients with acromegaly. The modern medical manual includes methods of surgical treatment, drug therapy and radiation exposure. Each of these options has variable effectiveness and specific side effects that must be taken into account when planning a medical program. The criteria for biochemical remission in the treatment of acromegaly are: the age-appropriate level of IGF-1, sporadic level of GH <1 mcg/l and the value of GH nadir when using OGTT with 75 g of glucose <0.4 mcg/l (when using a highly sensitive method for determining GH). Taking into account age and laboratory fluctuations of the normal values of the IGF-1, it is recommended to use a unified indicator of the IGF-1 index, reflecting the amount of excess of the IGF-1 above the upper limit of age norm (IGF-1 index = IGF-1/ULN), the target value of which should be <1. Unfortunately, in a number of national registries and retrospective studies, free handling of the remission target is practiced, in which an increase in the value of the IGF-1 index to 1.2 and 1.3 is allowed; which is not consistent with consensus agreements. Such artificial improvement of statistical indicators increases the rating of the register but negatively affects the therapeutic prognosis, since it eliminates the need for therapeutic correction. This remark also applies to the interpretation of cut-off points. It is clear that at different target values of acromegaly control (for example, at values IGF-1 index <1 or < 1.3), different indicators of cut-off points of prognostic independent variables are assumed, which complicates the development of a consolidated prognostic protocol. Therefore, when assessing the predictive power of the proposed predictors (or thresholds), it is necessary to additionally indicate the remission targets IGF-1 index used in a specific retrospective study [21, 22].

The purpose of this work is to discuss the priority of clinical and laboratory markers and the validation of independent variables that determine the prognosis of the effectiveness of therapeutic measures, including surgical aid and long-term use of first-generation somatostatin receptor ligands (fg-SRLs).

4. Predictors of the prospects and adequacy of surgical aid

According to international recommendations, transsphenoidal adenomectomy of somatotroph pituitary neuroendocrine tumor (PitNET) is the first-line treatment of acromegaly with a high chance of complete cure of the majority of patients with acromegaly. Pharmacological treatment is recommended if surgery is contraindicated or did not lead to disease remission. The choice of treatment best fitting each patient should be based on a thorough investigation of patients' characteristics.

4.1 Predictors of postoperative remission

The indicators of postoperative (p/o) biochemical remission vary from 32 to 85% depending on the size of the tumor, the severity of invasion of the cavernous sinus, the qualifications of the neurosurgeon and the control criteria used. With delayed diagnosis and large tumor sizes with suprasellar and parasellar growth, radical adenomectomy is possible only in 40–60% of cases. The ambiguity of surgical outcomes contributed to the development of a prognostic direction that determines the effectiveness of the planned surgical aid and the likelihood of adjuvant treatment. In addition to the dynamics of p/o hormonal parameters, among the clinical biomarkers that allow predicting the likelihood of remission, there are: initial indicators of hormonal and proliferative activity of tumor, its volume and the nature of extracellular spread, as well as radiological signs of invasive growth. Later, radiometric and immunophenotypic characteristics of somatotrophic tumors were added to the general list [23, 24].

Taweesomboonyat et al. showed that the remission rate after transsphenoidal removal of micro- and macroadenomas is 100 and 44%, respectively. The conducted multifactorial analysis showed that the combination of a high preoperative value of IGF-1 index (> 2.5) and the presence of 3–4 degrees of adenoma enlargement on the Knosp grade are unfavorable prognostic factors regarding the radicality of the upcoming surgery and indicate the need for subsequent adjuvant treatment [25].

In a retrospective study by Cardinal et al., it was shown that the preoperative level of IGF-1 and the value of GH on the first day after surgery are inversely correlated with hormonal remission. A drop in the concentration of GH in the first 1–2 days after surgery <1.55 ng/ml is a predictor of its success. At the same time, the sensitivity of this indicator, according to the authors, was 75, the specificity was 59%. The average sporadic GH level in patients who achieved remission was 1.6 versus 9.5 ng/ml in patients with persistent activity. In a similar work by Mohyeldin et al., it was found that the value of GH-nadir during OGTT 24–48 hours after surgery <1.15 ng/ml is the best predictor of remission with a sensitivity of 73% and specificity of 85%. As a result of the multivariate logistic regression analysis Tomasik et al. have established that such indicators, as a sporadic concentration of GH < 8.63, the maximum diameter < 15.5 mm, the presence of normoprolactinemia, DGST, positive staining on α-SU на are independent predictors of surgical remission [26–28].

Since no single marker is able to independently predict the postoperative outcome, prognostic models and nomograms are usually used, including a complex of diverse predictors and allowing to significantly increase their sensitivity and specificity. In the work of Agrawal et al., a mathematical analysis of retrospective studies with the identification of factors affecting the effectiveness of the surgical intervention is presented. It was noted that the young age of patients, a large tumor volume, initially high levels of GH and IGF-1 and the presence of signs of invasion of the cavernous sinus may be predictors of non-radical adenomectomy [29].

Heng et al. proposed a predictive model that allows predicting the presence of SGST with a high degree of probability, characterized by aggressive behavior and a tendency to relapse. The study included 44 patients with DGST and 39 patients with SGST. In the course of comparing the data of the preoperative examination with the results of the morphological diagnosis, it was found that patients with SGST were distinguished by a young age, large adenoma sizes, a high degree of invasion and low sensitivity to octreotide treatment. Thus, the size of the tumor, the degree of invasion on the Knosp scale, the value of the GH index and the percentage of decrease in GH against the background of octreotide administration are independent variables, the combination of which made it possible to compile a graduated scale for predicting SGST with an AUC value of 0.84 and high sensitivity and specificity. According to Swanson et al., the absence of invasion and lower pre-operative IGF-1 index were the only significant predictors of post-surgical remission in this cohort [30, 31].

4.2 Predictors of recurrence or continued growth of a residual tumor

A separate topic is the prediction of the risk of the continued growth of a residual tumor and/or relapse, which seems to be important for determining the strategy of active dynamic control. According to the data presented by Lucas et al., continued growth is observed in 12–58% of patients with residual tumors. Even with radical adenomectomy, 10–20% of operated patients have a relapse of the disease over the next 5–10 years. It is noted that the very fact of the presence of residual tissue is the leading condition for continued growth. According to observations, the overall recurrence rate after 5, 10 and 15 years was 25%, 43% and 61%, respectively. At the same time, an inverse correlation was found between the patient's age and the risk of further growth of residual tissue. It was also shown that the risk of p/o growth of the remaining tissue outside the sella turcica was 3.7 times higher than that of resident tumors confined to the sella turcica area. Therefore, more active treatment strategies should be used for patients with extrasellar tumor tissue residue [32]. In the process of conducting logistic regression analysis, Mohyeldin et al. identified three statistically significant independent variables indicating a high risk of invasion of the medial wall of the cavernous sinus: the degree of tumor enlargement on the Knosp scale >2; male sex; the presence of an aggressive form of somatotrophic tumor [27].

A clinical study by Freda et al. is of interest, according to the results of which it is concluded that the risk of p/o relapse increases in persons with achieved normalization of IGF-1, but impaired suppression of GH against the background of OGTT. Thus, the pathological value of the GH-nadir may indicate the presence of an autonomous formation [33].

In the prognostic model of continued tumor growth L. Lu et al suggest including markers such as the young age of patients; high pre-operative level of secretory activity; signs of invasive growth; volume and localization of residual tissue; preservation of pseudocapsules; presence of aggressive morphological subtype (SGST) [23].

In the work of Wang et al., 178 patients with pituitary adenomas were retrospectively analyzed with the release of predictors indicating a high level of Ki-67 (>3%). In the process of multivariate regression analysis, it was shown that young age, the abundant blood supply to the tumor and erosion of the back of the turcica sella are independent markers of a high value of the proliferative index Ki-67, and, consequently, the risk of residual growth. In a study by Chen et al., it was noted that independent factors such as BMI (> 25 kg/m2), the 4th degree of increase on the Knosp scale, partial resection, Ki-67 (>3%) can serve as predictors of postoperative progression of tumor growth or recurrence of pituitary adenomas [34, 35].

On the contrary, the predictor of a low risk of relapse is: older age, small tumor, low level of secretory activity, benign morphological subtype, postoperative radiation therapy. According to Lu et al., the recurrence rate in patients who did not receive radiation therapy increased progressively during the follow-up period, reaching 72% after 15 years. On the contrary, in patients who received timely radiotherapy, the recurrence rate stabilized at 9% after 10 years [23].

Thus, these data indicate the practical importance of improving prognostic models that allow determining the postoperative scenario of the disease and the need for adjuvant therapy.

5. Predictors of sensitivity to somatostatin receptor ligands

The existing problem of drug therapy (DT) acromegaly is the lack of a differentiated approach when choosing a targeted drug, taking into account the receptor phenotype of a somatotrophic tumor. Its solution is connected with the identification and verification of clinical and biological predictors that allow identifying groups of patients sensitive to the planned treatment [36]. Current pharmacological options for patients with acromegaly include somatostatin receptor ligands (SRLs), growth hormone receptor agonists, and dopamine agonists (DA). Somatostatin receptor ligands (SRLs) have been used in clinical practice for more than 30 years and play a leading role in the treatment of acromegaly. Currently, three extended forms of SRLs are widely used worldwide (octreotide, lanreotide and pasireotide), which occupy an important place in the algorithm of treatment of acromegaly. It is known that the cells of somatotropic adenomas mainly contain the 2nd and 5th subtypes of somatostatin receptors (SSTRs), the intensity of membrane expression of which is a key factor in the implementation of the suppressive action of SRLs. By acting on the somatostatin receptors of adenomatous cells, SRLs provide a dose-dependent blockade of the rhythmic secretion of GH and inhibition of cell growth.

The binding of SRLs to SSTRs promotes the dissociation of the Gi protein receptor complex, followed by a decrease in the activity of adenylate cyclase, leading to the opening of potassium channels, hyperpolarization of the cell membrane and closure of calcium channels. The changes in ion permeability resulting from the activation of the receptor lead to a critical decrease in the intracellular concentration of calcium ions and cAMP, which blocks the secretion of GH and the proliferation of somatotrophs. Activation of SSTRs and specific proteins involved in intracellular signal transmission (AIP, ZAC1, RKIP, E-cadherin, β-arrestin) promotes suppression of GH secretion, inhibition of proliferation, cell migration and angiogenesis [16, 19, 37].

The prevalent expression of SSTR2 in GH-secreting adenomas makes it a prime target for treating acromegaly. The first-generation SRLs (fg-SRLs) (octreotide LAR and lanreotide autogel) preferentially bind to SSTR2, thereby suppressing GH expression. The introduction of these drugs into wide clinical practice has significantly increased the effectiveness of acromegaly treatment and the quality of life of patients. Comparative results of the use of prolonged forms of octreotide and lanreotide in patients with acromegaly showed similar characteristics. In the work of Albarel et al., a meta-analysis of the effectiveness of treatment of fg-SRLs in 4464 patients with acromegaly was carried out, during which normalization of levels of GH and IGF-1 was noted in 56 and 55% of patients, respectively [18, 38, 39].

The second important option of the therapeutic effect of SRLs is their antitumor effect due to the development of apoptosis and necrosis of tumor cells. Confirmation of the anti-proliferative effect of SRLs is in vivo studies, which revealed lower indicators of the proliferative index Ki-67 in somatotrophic tumor tissue obtained from patients who were previously treated with octreotide, compared with naive patients [40].

The presence of a direct correlation between the expression of the SSTR2 in adenomatous cells, on the one hand, and the degree of decrease in tumor volume, as well as the severity of biochemical sensitivity to the LAR octreotide, on the other hand, was revealed. According to A. Colao et al., the greatest decrease in volume (about 50% of the initial one) is observed during the 1st year of treatment. During the PRIMARY clinical trial, it was noted that 63% of patients receiving lanreotide Autogel achieved a significant (> 20%) reduction in tumor volume within 48 weeks. At the same time, the magnitude of the decrease in the level of IGF-1 during treatment was the most significant predictor of a decrease in tumor mass. A decrease in the volume of the tumor by more than 20% from the initial one was observed in 66% of patients receiving octreotide LAR (an average decrease of 51%) and in 63% of patients receiving Lanreotide Autogel (an average decrease of 27%). The study of Albarel et al. included a cohort of 1685 patients. Meta-analysis of the results of 41 clinical studies revealed a decrease in the volume of tumors (by an average of 50.6%) in 66% of patients with primary DT fg-SRLs [39, 41, 42]. Biomarkers a guiding a more precise therapy.

Clinical practice has shown that fg-SRLs have a good safety profile, with the most common side effects being mild gastrointestinal symptoms observed in 30% of patients and rarely leading to discontinuation of the drug. Mild hyperglycemia was observed in 15% of patients, and cholelithiasis was observed in 35% of patients treated with fg-SRLs for more than 3–6 months [19, 39].

5.1 The phenomenon of resistance to fg-SRLs

Nevertheless, the results of a long-term study showed that the effectiveness of using fg-SRLs in a non-selective sample, according to various authors, does not exceed 50–55%. In a prospective study evaluating the effectiveness of lanreotide (120 mg every 28 days) as a first-line therapy, it was shown that the normalization of GH levels and IGF-I after 24 and 48 weeks of treatment were observed in 23.4 and 30.6% of patients. Thus, a significant part of patients receiving fg-SRLs has partial or complete resistance, which is a consequence of the internal heterogeneity of somatotropin in relation to the receptor expression of SSTs and other target molecules affecting the therapeutic response [16–18].

It should be noted that, according to consensus agreements, prolonged forms of fg-SRLs are the starting drug therapy, while other medicinal preparations are prescribed with fatal delay and only after realizing the obvious ineffectiveness of long-term pharmacotherapy. Modest results of fg-SRLs treatment are the expected result of a non-personalized approach, when with the help of a single drug the doctor tries to cure all morphotypes of somatotrophic tumors, including those with a different receptor phenotype. The traditional answer to the detected low sensitivity to fg-SRLs is an escalation of the dose of the drug (or a reduction in injection intervals), followed by the connection of a 2nd-line drug—a selective dopamine agonist (cabergoline). Switching to taking drugs with a different mechanism of action is recommended to be done no earlier than after 12 months of DT. According to Kasuki et al., despite the maximum doses of the drug and the long duration of treatment of fg-SRLs, 20–25% of patients retain the activity of the disease, fraught with the progressive development of multiple organ disorders [43, 44].

A more successful therapeutic practice in detecting resistance to fg-SRLs is switching to a multiligand analog of somatostatin of the 2nd generation of long-acting—pasyreotide LAR, which, unlike octreotide, has half the affinity for the SSTR2 and a higher (5 and 40 times) affinity for the SSTR3 and SSTR5. It shows more efficacious in patients resistant to fg-SRLs.

It is noted that in real clinical practice, biochemical remission against the background of treatment with pasireotide LAR is achieved in approximately 54% of patients resistant to fg-SRLs. A decrease in tumor volume (≥ 20%) was observed in 80.8% of pasireotide LAR and in 77.4% of patients receiving octreotide LAR. At the same time, there is a correlation between the sensitivity to pasireotide and the increased intensity of the MR signal in T2-weighted images [45–47].

Unfortunately, despite the high antisecretory and antitumor activity, taking this drug in about 60% of cases is accompanied by a violation of carbohydrate metabolism, which limits its clinical use outside the resistant group. Further development of multiligand drugs will allow to unify pharmacotherapy of various subtypes of somatotrophic tumors. In this regard, great hopes are pinned on the drug Veldoreotide (Somatropim) undergoing clinical trials, which has a lower hyperglycemic effect [19, 37].

A selective agonist of dopaminergic receptors, cabergoline (CAB) represents another therapeutic option in acromegaly, but their efficacy to control GH secretion is not related to the degree of DRD2 expression in somatotrophic tumors. Pharmacological niches of cabergoline use are: a/small disease activity (IGF-1 index<2), b/presence of mixed somato-lactotrophic tumors, c/detection of partial resistance to fg-SRLs as a 2nd-line drug. As monotherapy, cabergoline is effective in 20–30% of cases. In case of partial resistance to SRLs, the addition of CAB to SRLs is an option and can lead to IGF-1 normalization in 50% of additional patients [37, 48, 49].

Another pharmacological option for detecting resistance (or non-tolerance) of fg-SRLs is the appointment of a GH receptor antagonist—a pegvisomant, that blocks the biological effect of GH in peripheral tissues (primarily in the liver). The drug does not affect tumor activity and blocks the biological effect of GH, steadfastly normalizing the level of IGF-1 in the blood in 63–97% of cases. Pegvisomant (Somavert) can be used as monotherapy (for small adenoma sizes) or in combination with SRLs (or CAB). The 14-year observation program ACROSTUDY, which brought together 2221 patients from different countries, showed the presence of persistent biochemical control in 72% of patients with acromegaly. The continued growth of residual adenoma was observed in 3.7% of patients. For patients with initially high hormonal activity (IGF-1 index >2.7), diabetes mellitus, increased body mass index (>30 kg/m2), higher starting doses and accelerated titration of the preparation are required to normalize IGF-1 [50, 51].

The indication for the appointment of pegvisomant is the preservation of the activity of the disease after nonradical adenomectomy and ineffective secondary DT. The combination with pegvisomant in patients with partial response to fg-SRLs allows disease control in 80% of patients. The advantages of combination therapy include higher efficiency with lower doses of pegvisomant, as well as stabilization of the size of residual tissue. Thus, thanks to the appearance of pasireotide and pegvisomant, an additional therapeutic maneuver became possible to achieve control, but fg-SRLs, as before, occupy leading positions in the drug treatment of acromegaly [19, 21, 52].

The gold standard for determining the drug strategy of secondary DT is the molecular phenotyping of fragments of a removed tumor using immunohistochemical (IHC) analysis). Depending on the morphotype of the somatotrophic tumor, there is a characteristic difference in receptor expression. Thus, DGST predominantly expresses the SSTR2, whereas SGST, certain types of somato-lactotrophic tumors and low—differentiated forms—mainly the SSTR5, which indicates the possibility of differentiated DT acromegaly taking into account the receptor phenotype.

5.2 Predictors of sensitivity to fg-SRLs

The recognition of the fact of the multiplicity of pathomorphological variants of somatotrophic tumors contributed to the development of tumor-oriented diagnostics by determining predictors indicating the presence of a certain morphotype and a feature of receptor expression, including evaluation samples with octreotide and signifor, secretory and morphological characteristics of the tumor, the results of IHC analysis and the intensity of the tumor signal on T2-weighted MR images. Among the predictors of sensitivity to fg-SRLs are: female sex, older age, a slight excess of the levels of GH and IGF-1, the presence of *GNAS* mutation and DGST, high expression of the SSTR2, a low value of the proliferative index Ki-67, pronounced response to an acute test with octreotide, as well as the detection of hypointensive adenoma on T2-weighted MR images. On the contrary, in young male patients with a high level of GH at diagnosis, the presence of *AIP* mutation, SGST and hyperintensive tumor signal on T2-weighted images are associated with low sensitivity to fg-SRLs. It is also noted that miRNAs might influence tumor proliferation, invasion, size, and response to fg-SRLs [18, 19, 24, 34, 53, 54].

Although not routinely evaluated by clinical pathologists, SST expression may be a valuable molecular marker for precision-based acromegaly treatment, as a decision for repeat surgery, radiotherapy or choice of a specific SRL could be better guided with a knowledge of SSTR2 and SSTR5 expression According to Störmann et al. the best results of 12-month treatment of fg-SRLs were observed in patients older than 53 years, female, with high expression of the SSTR2. In the study of Durmus et al., it was shown that older passport age, low initial levels of GH and IGF-1 at the time of diagnosis, small tumor volume, hypo-intensity signal on T2-weighted MR images and the presence of densely granular adenoma allow predicting a good biochemical response to fg-SRLs [16, 55, 56].

Puig-Domingo et al. suggest that when choosing a treatment strategy, focus on the data of the intensity of the tumor signal on T2-weighted MR images in combination with the results of acute tests with octreotide and pasireotide, which makes it more likely to determine the most promising candidate. The author believes that the development of an acute pasireotide test will be of much aid in the context of personalized medicine [57].

Coopmans et al. multivariable regression models for predicting the biochemical response to fg-SRLs was proposed. In this study, the biochemical response was categorized as follows: biochemical response (IGF-I ≤ 1.3 ULN), partial response (>20% relative IGF-I reduction without normalization) and nonresponse (≤ 20% relative IGF-I reduction). As a result of a meta-analysis of 622 patients, it was shown that low baseline IGF-I levels and low body weight were the best independent predictors of the biochemical response to first-generation SRLs [AUC 0.77 (95% CI, 0.72–0.81)] [58].

In a retrospective analysis of the treatment results of 153 acromegaly patients by Tomasik et al., it was shown that the older age of diagnosis, male gender, low concentrations of GH, IGF-1 and prolactin, small tumor size, as well as the presence of a-SU, low index Ki-67 and DGST are the best independent predictors of good response to fg-SRLs. The cut-off value of fasting GH concentration predicting good response to fg-SRLs was estimated as GH < 36.6 μg/L with a sensitivity of 45.5% and specificity of 80.0%. The percentage of correctly classified patients was 52.4%. The AUC value was 0,788 [28].

The predictor algorithm of resistance to octreotide (and sensitivity to pasireotide) proposed by a number of authors includes: young age, male sex, large tumor size, high secretory activity, presence of SGST, high membrane expression SSTR5, low ratio between the SSTR2 and SSTR5, as well as low expression of zinc finger protein (ZAC1) regulating apoptosis and cell cycle arrest. Thus, molecular genotyping and identification of clinical and pathological markers are necessary tools for selecting the optimal therapeutic drug [59–61].

Kasuki et al. noted that high Ki-67 values (2.3% cut-off point) correlate with low sensitivity of fg-SRLs. The Ki-67 level was higher in SGST compared to DGST (p = 0.047). It was also shown that higher expression of the SSTR2 and the presence of DGST significantly correlated with sensitivity to fg-SRLs. The authors conclude that the value of Ki-67, as well as the expression of the SSTR2, can be independent predictors of the effectiveness of using fg-SRLs. During the regression analysis conducted by Gill et al., it was noted that the most significant prognostic biomarker determining sensitivity to fg-SRLs is E-cadherin, whose sensitivity was 73%. The second most important independent factor was the expression of the SSTR2. The combination of these 2 predictors increased the accuracy of the forecast by up to 80%. Thus, low expression of E-cadherin is a marker not only of aggressive behavior of the tumor but also of resistance to fg-SRLs. In a study by Puig-Domingo et al., the predictive value of E-cadherine, SSTR2 and Ki-67 was also confirmed [18, 62, 63].

5.3 Pharmacotherapeutic testing

It should be noted that in modern consensus agreements, fg-SRLs are recommended to all patients (without taking into account morphological diagnosis) as secondary or primary pharmacotherapy by "trial and error". Since sensitivity to fg-SRLs, according to various authors, is observed in 40–50% of cases, it is not surprising that in some patients this appointment will be obviously ineffective due to a fundamentally different receptor phenotype of tumor cells. Hence, the question arises, what should be the optimal duration of trial treatment of fg-SRLs during traditional therapy in order to predict their long-term effectiveness?

To answer this question, we conducted a comparative analysis of the effectiveness of long-term primary (1) and secondary (2) DT fg-SRLs among 587 patients included in the Moscow Registry of Patients with Acromegaly, during which it was shown that in the selective group (with a decrease in IGF-1 of more than 70% of the baseline level after 3 months of treatment) biochemical remission was observed in 72 and 80% of cases compared with 47 and 51% in the non-selective group (p = 0.0002). The correlation coefficients between the percentage of reduction of IGF-1 after 3 months of treatment and dynamic indicators are presented in **Table 1** (p = 0.000). These data indicate the practical importance of the selective selection of patients for the treatment of fg-SRLs [64].

		IGF-1 after 12 months (ng/ml)	IGF-1 at the end of treatment (ng/ml)	Duration of effective treatment (months)
% reduction of IGF-1 after 3 months of treatment fg-SRLs	1 DT	−0,57	−0,61	0,52
	2 DT	−0,51	−0,43	0,43

Table 1.
Correlation analysis of the long-term effectiveness of fg-SRLs depending on the severity of the decrease in IGF-1 3 months after the start of treatment.

In the subsequent work, a retrospective clinical and morphological comparison was carried out, which included 33 (12 men) patients with DGST and 47 (17 men) patients with SGST. The age of diagnosis was 48.4 ± 11.4 vs. 39.4 ± 12.7 years ($p = 0.0027$), the volume of the residual tumor was 1.6 ± 3.5 vs. 2.7 ± 4.8 cm^3 ($p = 0.2$), the value of IGF-1 index before DT was 2.8 ± 0.8 vs. 2.7 + 0.9 ($p = 0.6$), respectively, [M(s)]. In the treatment, prolonged forms of lanreotide (Somatulin Autogel, s/c, 120 mg/28–56 days) or octreotide (Octreotide Depot, Octreotide Long, i/m at a dose of 10–30 mg/28 days) were used. The duration of DT was 21.5 ± 21.8 months. The adequacy of pharmacotherapy was assessed by the value IGF-1 index ≤1,0. The control points of pharmacotherapeutic testing were IGF-1 indicators before DT, as well as after 3, 6, 12 months of treatment and at the last visit.

The analysis confirmed good sensitivity to fg-SRLs in patients with DGST compared to SGST. The final value of IGF-1 index was 0.95 ± 0.27 vs. 1.4 ± 0.64 ($p = 0.0002$) (**Figure 1**).

It was noted that the percentage of decrease in IGF-1 after 3 and 6 months of fg-SRLs treatment compared to the baseline level directly correlates with the number of SSTR2 according to the IRS ($r = 0.44$; $r = 0.36$), as well as the difference and the ratio between the SSTR2 and SSTR5 [$r = 0.46$; $r = 0.46$ and $r = 0.41$; $r = 0.43$; ($p < 0.05$)]. Against the background of fg-SRLs treatment, the decrease in the level of IGF-1 in the groups of patients with DGST and SGST after 3 months was 54.8 ± 19.6 vs. 28.4 ± 23.7%, after 6 months—58.4 ± 18.0 vs. 31.6 ± 24.5%, respectively ($p = 0.0002$). The presence of an inverse correlation was revealed between the indicators of a decrease in the level of IGF-1 after 3 and 6 months of fg-SRLs treatment and the final value of IGF-1 index [$r = -0.59$; and $r = -0.72$; ($p < 0.001$)]. According to the results of the ROC analysis, the AUC was 0.841 and 0.853, respectively, which confirms the good informative value of the selected diagnostic indicators. Cut-off prognostic points of effective DT were a decrease in the level of IGF-1 after 3 and 6 months to 46 and 49%, the sensitivity of these markers was 63 and 75% and specificity—79 and 80% (**Figure 2**). With a decrease in the level of IGF-1 after 3 and 6 months of less than 50%, the final IGF-1 index was 1.49 ± 0.62, whereas with a decrease of more than 50%, the average value of IGF-1 index in the long-term treatment of fg-SRLs was

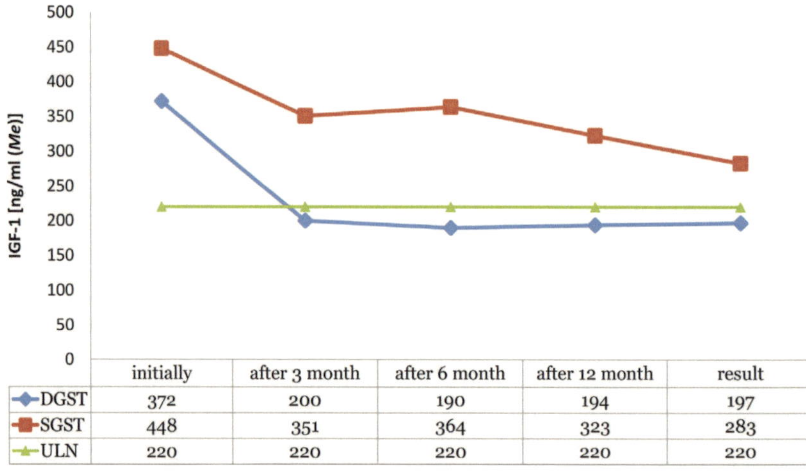

	initially	after 3 month	after 6 month	after 12 month	result
DGST	372	200	190	194	197
SGST	448	351	364	323	283
ULN	220	220	220	220	220

Figure 1.
Dynamics of IGF-1 level against the background of fg-SRLs treatment of patients with DGST and SGST.

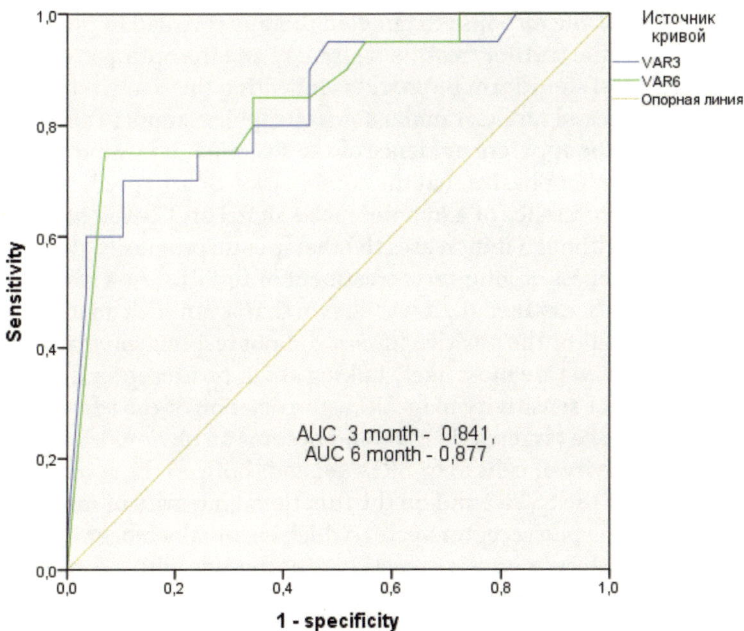

Figure 2.
Significance of prognostic model of the reduction IGF-1 after 3 and 6 months of fg-SRLs treatment.

0.9 ± 0.2; (p = 0.000). [Later, pegvisomant with a positive effect was added to the treatment of resistant patients with SGST. IGF-1 index decreased to 0.98 + 0.44].

The data obtained confirm that the nature of the decrease in IGF-1 from the baseline level after 3 and 6 months of treatment reflects the severity of absolute or relative overexpression of the SSTR2 in tumor cells, and also indicates the intact postreceptor suppressive mechanisms. Thus, the results of pharmacotherapeutic testing can be used as an additional predictor of the effectiveness of long-term treatment of fg-SRLs and the determination of optimal therapeutic tactics to achieve stable control of acromegaly [65].

This conclusion is consistent with the data provided by M.R. Gadelha et al., who noted that the expression of mRNA of the SSTR2 correlated with a decrease in the levels of GH and IGF-1 after 3 and 6 months of octreotide treatment, as well as with a decrease in tumor volume. It was also noted that in the presence of DGST, the chances of a good response to fg-SRLs were more than 10 times higher than with SGST [19, 28].

Returning to the topic of precision medicine, it should be noted that the main limitation of the use of biomarkers for predicting the effectiveness of DT is the small number of patients included in the studies and the lack of unified methods for analyzing the expression of SSTR2 and other characteristics of tumor cells, which makes it difficult to interpret the results. According to M.R. Gadelha, it is time to change the paradigm of secondary DT by prescribing differentiated treatment taking into account the postoperative hormonal status and expression of SSTR2, SSTR5, AIP and DR2 in tumor cells [19].

In our opinion, the leading system-forming factor that allows the stratification of various clinical and pathological markers is a specific morphological subtype of somatotrophic adenoma, which should become a predictor of the 1st degree, reflecting the features of the biological functioning of autonomous tumor cells with more or less predictable behavior. The immunotypic characteristics, indicators of mitotic activity and features of the response to targeted therapy revealed in this case make it possible to determine the further treatment strategy and the optimal scheme of DT. **Table 2** shows the most significant biomarkers reflecting the characteristics of the most common densely and rarely granular somatotrophic tumors (**Table 2**).

However, with all the apparent evidence of the situation, it is impossible not to mention the works that emphasize that the combination of sign predictors (expression of the SSTR2, the presence of a hypointensive signal on T2-weighted MRI, detection of DGST), although it increases the therapeutic prognosis, does not yet guarantee the effectiveness of long-term treatment of fg-SRLs. As a result of a meta-analysis conducted by S. Ezzat et al., it was shown that, even with good expression of the SSTR2, about half of the positive tumors did not respond clinically to fg-SRLs [66]. Since in this case, we are most likely talking about postreceptor disorders, then, among the predictors of sensitivity to fg-SRLs, the reaction of the adenoma itself to the administration of a targeted drug should become an obvious biomarker. It is known that the sensitivity of cells to fg-SRLs depends both on the severity of the receptor expression of the SSTR2 and on the functional integrity of multiple intracellular components of the postreceptor vector, which eventually blocks the pathological secretion of GH. Therefore, a positive reaction to octreotide with a marked decrease in the level of GH (and, accordingly, IGF-1) allows us to judge the complex integrity

Predictors	**DGST**	**SGST**
Age of debut of acromegaly	more than 40 years	less than 40 years old
Tumor size	micro-, macroadenomas	macro-, giant adenomas
Localization of the tumor	intrasellar location	extrasellar distribution
Invasion of the cavernous sinus	not typical	typical, 3-4 gr Knosp
The tendency to residual growth and recurrence of the tumor	low	high
Intensity of the tumor signal on T2-weighted magnetic imaging	hypointensive	hyperintensive
Expression of the SSTR2	high	low
Expression of the SSTR5	low	high
Evaluation test with octreotide	positive	negative
Sensitivity to fg-SRLs	high	low
Reduction of IGF-1 after 3 and 6 months of treatment fg-SRLs	> 50%	< 50%
Proliferation index Ki-67	low (<3%)	high (>3%)
Expression of the α-subunit	high	absent
Cytokeratin expression	low	high
Expression E-cadherin	high	low
Expression ZAC1		
GNAS-mutationis	positive	negative
AIP-mutationis	negative	positive

Table 2.
Clinical and biological predictors of DGST and SGST.

of the receptor and postreceptor mechanisms and, accordingly, the prospects of the planned long-term drug therapy.

Precision medicine aims to improve patient outcomes through targeted treatment employing genetic, biomarker, phenotypic, or psychosocial characteristics unique to each patient or the disease process. Of course, radiological and/or IHC confirmation of the presence of DGST is extremely important for determining the benign nature of the clinical course of adenoma but does not guarantee absolute sensitivity to fg-SRLs. Therefore, in our opinion, additional predictors of successful lifelong therapy of fg-SRLs should be the results of pharmacotherapeutic testing determining a more accurate treatment strategy. This tactic also allows timely identification of a group of patients with fg-SRLs resistance and aggressive course of the disease who need fundamentally different treatment.

Author details

Vyacheslav S. Pronin[1,2]*, Mikhail B. Antsiferov[1,2], Tatyana M. Alekseeva[2] and Evgeny V. Pronin[2]

1 Federal State Budgetary Educational Institution, Additional Professional Education, Russian Medical Academy of Continuing Professional Education, The Ministry of Health of the Russian Federation, Moscow, Russia

2 The Moscow Health Department, Moscow Endocrinology Dispensary, State Budgetary Healthcare Institute, Moscow, Russia

*Address all correspondence to: vspronin@yandex.ru

References

[1] Gadelha MR, Kasuki L, Lim DS, Fleseriu M. Systemic complications of acromegaly and the impact of the current treatment landscape: An update. Endocrine Reviews. 2019;**40**:268-232. DOI: 10.1210/er.2018-00115

[2] Esposito D et al. Prolonged diagnostic delay in acromegaly is associated with increased morbidity and mortality. European Journal of Endocrinology. 2020;**182**(6):523-531

[3] Caron P. Signs and symptoms of acromegaly at diagnosis: The physician's and the patient's perspectives in the ACRO-POLIS study. Endocrine. 2019;**63**(1):120-129

[4] Lavrentaki A, Paluzzi A, Wass JAH, Karavitaki N. Epidemiology of acromegaly: Review of population studies. Pituitary. 2017;**20**(1):4-9. DOI: 10.1007/s11102-016-0754-x

[5] Zarool-Hassan R et al. Symptoms and signs of acromegaly: An ongoing need to raise awareness among healthcare practitioners. Journal of Primary Health Care. 2016;**8**(2):157-163

[6] Sisco J, van der Lely AJ. Towards an earlier diagnosis of acromegaly and gigantism. Journal of Clinical Medicine. 2021;**10**(7):1363

[7] Meng T et al. Identifying facial features and predicting patients of acromegaly using three-dimensional imaging techniques and machine learning. Frontiers in Endocrinology (Lausanne). 2020;**11**:492

[8] Asa SL, Kucharczyk W, Ezzat S. Pituitary acromegaly: Not one disease. Endocrine-Related Cancer. 2017;**24**(3):C1-C4. DOI: 10.1530/ERC-16-0496

[9] Asa SL, Ezzat S. An update on pituitary neuroendocrine tumors leading to acromegaly and gigantism. Journal of Clinical Medicine. 2021;**10**(11):2254. DOI: 10.3390/jcm10112254

[10] Lopes M.B.S. The 2017 World Health Organization classification of tumors of the pituitary gland: A summary Acta Neuropathologica 2017. Vol. 134, N 4. P. 521-535. doi: 10.1007/s00401-017-1769-8

[11] Asa SL, Mete O, Perry A, Osamura RY. Overview of the 2022 WHO classification of pituitary tumors. Endocrine Pathology. 2022;**33**(1):6-26. DOI: 10.1007/s12022-022-09703-7

[12] Mete O, Lopes MB. Overview of the 2017 WHO classification of pituitary tumors. Endocrine Pathology. 2017;**28**:228-243. DOI: 10.1007/s12022-017-9498-z

[13] Akirov A, Asa SL, Amer L, Shimon I, et al. The Clinicopathological Spectrum of acromegaly. Journal of Clinical Medicine. 2019;**8**(11):1962. DOI: 10.3390/jcm8111962

[14] Trouillas J, Jaffrain-Rea M-L, Vasiljevic A, Dekkers O, et al. Are aggressive pituitary tumors and carcinomas two sides of the same coin? Pathologists reply to clinician's questions. Reviews in Endocrine & Metabolic Disorders 2020. Vol. 21, N 2. P. 243-251. doi: 10.1007/s11154-020-09562-9

[15] Chang M, Yang C, Bao X, Wang R. Genetic and epigenetic causes of pituitary adenomas. Frontiers Endocrinology (Lausanne). 2020;**11**:596554. DOI: 10.3389/fendo.2020.596554

[16] Labadzhyan A, Melmed S. Molecular targets in acromegaly. Front Endocrinol

(Lausanne). 2022;**5**(13):1068061. DOI: 10.3389/fendo.2022.1068061

[17] Ku CR., Melnikov V, Zhang Z, Lee EJ. Precision therapy in acromegaly caused by pituitary tumors: How close is it to reality? Endocrinology and Metabolism (Seoul). 2020; Vol. 35, N 2. P. 206-216. doi: 10.3803/EnM.2020.35.2.206

[18] Puig-Domingo M, Gil J, Sampedro-Nunez M, Jorda M, et al. Molecular profiling for acromegaly treatment: A validation study. Endocrine-Related Cancer. 2020;**27**(6):375-389. DOI: 10.1530/ERC-18-0565

[19] Gadelha M.R., Wildemberg L.E., Kasuki L. The future of somatostatin receptor ligands in acromegaly. The Journal of Clinical Endocrinology and Metabolism 2022, Vol. 107, N 2. P. 297-308. doi: 10.1210/clinem/dgab726

[20] Nista F, Corica G, Castelletti L, Khorrami K, Campana C, et al. Clinical and radiological predictors of biochemical response to first-line treatment with somatostatin receptor ligands in acromegaly: A real-life perspective. Frontiers in Endocrinology (Lausanne). 2021;**12**:677919. DOI: 10.3389/fendo.2021.677919

[21] Fleseriu M, Biller BMK, Freda PU, Gadelha MR, et al. A pituitary society update to acromegaly management guidelines. Pituitary, 2021. Vol. *24*, N 1. P. 1-13. doi: 10.1007/s11102-020-01091-7

[22] Liu C-X, Wang S-Z, Heng L-J, Han Y, et al. Predicting subtype of growth hormone pituitary adenoma based on magnetic resonance imaging characteristics. Journal of Computer Assisted Tomography 2022. Vol. 46, N 1. P. 124-130. doi: 10.1097/RCT.0000000000001249

[23] Lu L, Wan X, Xu Y, Chen J, et al. Development and validation of a prognostic model for post-operative recurrence of pituitary adenomas. Frontiers in Oncology. 2022;**12**:882049. DOI: 10.3389/fonc.2022.882049

[24] Dai C, Fan Y, Li Y, Bao X, et al. Development and interpretation of multiple machine learning models for predicting postoperative delayed remission of acromegaly patients during long-term follow-up. Frontiers in Endocrinology (Lausanne). 2020;**11**:643. DOI: 10.3389/fendo.2020.00643

[25] Taweesomboonyat C, Oearsakul T. Prognostic factors of Acromegalic patients with growth hormone-secreting pituitary adenoma after Transsphenoidal surgery. World Neurosurgery. 2021;**146**:e1360-e1366. DOI: 10.1016/j.wneu.2020.12.013

[26] Cardinal T, Collet C, Wedemeyer M, Singer PA, et al. Postoperative GH and degree of reduction in IGF-1 predicts postoperative hormonal remission in acromegaly. Frontiers in Endocrinology (Lausanne). 2021;**12**:743052. DOI: 10.3389/fendo.2021.743052

[27] Mohyeldin A, Katznelson LE, Hoffman AR, Asmaro K, et al. Prospective intraoperative and histologic evaluation of cavernous sinus medial wall invasion by pituitary adenomas and its implications for acromegaly remission outcomes. Scientific Reports 2022; Vol. 12, N 1. 9919. doi: 10.1038/s41598-022-12980-1

[28] Tomasik A, Stelmachowska-Banas M, Maksymowicz M, Czajka-Oraniec I, et al. Clinical, hormonal and pathomorphological markers of somatotroph pituitary neuroendocrine tumors predicting the treatment outcome in acromegaly. Frontiers in Endocrinology (Lausanne). 2022;**13**:957301. DOI: 10.3389/fendo.2022.957301

[29] Agraval N, Ioachimescu AC. Prognostic factors of biochemical remission after transsphenoidal surgery for acromegaly: A structured review. Pituitary 2020; Vol. 23, N 5. P. 582-594. doi: 10.1007/s11102-020-01063-x

[30] Heng L, Liu X, Guo W, Zhang S, et al. Preoperative prediction of granulation pattern subtypes in GH-secreting pituitary adenomas. Clinical Endocrinology 2021, Vol. 95, N 1. P. 134-142. doi: 10.1111/cen.14465

[31] Swanson AA, Erickson D, Donegan DM, Jenkins SM, et al. Clinical, biological, radiological, and pathological comparison of sparsely and densely granulated somatotroph adenomas: A single center experience from a cohort of 131 patients with acromegaly. Pituitary 2021. Vol. 24, N 2. P. 192-206. doi: 10.1007/s11102-020-01096-2

[32] Lucas JW, Bodach ME, Tumialan LM, Oyesiku NM, et al. Congress of Neurological Surgeons systematic review and evidence-based guideline on primary Management of Patients with Nonfunctioning Pituitary Adenomas. Neurosurgery. 2016;**79**:E533-E535. DOI: 10.1227/NEU.0000000000001389

[33] Freda PU, Bruce JN, Reyes-Vidal C, Singh S, et al. Prognostic value of nadir GH levels for long-term biochemical remission or recurrence in surgically treated acromegaly. Pituitary 2021. Vol. 24, N 2. P. 170-183. DOI: 10.1007/s11102-020-01094-4

[34] Wang M, Shen M, He W, Yang Y, et al. The value of an acute octreotide suppression test in predicting short-term efficacy of somatostatin analogues in acromegaly. Endocrine Journal 2016. Vol. 63, N 9. P. 819-834. doi: 10.1507/endocrj.EJ16-0175

[35] Chen Y, Cai F, Cao J, Gao F, et al. Progression after Transnasal sphenoidal surgical treatment of large and Giant pituitary adenomas and establish a nomogram to predict tumor prognosis. Frontiers in Endocrinology (Lausanne). 2021;**12**:793337. DOI: 10.3389/fendo.2021.793337

[36] Gomes-Porras M, Cardenas-Salas J, Alvares-Escola. Somatostatin analogs in clinical practice. A review. International Journal of Molecular Sciences. 2020;**21**(5):1682. DOI: 10.3390/ijms21051682

[37] Sahakian N, Castinetti F, Brue T, Cuny T. Current and emerging medical therapies in pituitary tumors. Journal of Clinical Medicine. 2022;**11**(4):955. DOI: 10.3390/jcm11040955

[38] Liu W, Xie L, He M, Shen M, Zhu J, Yang Y, et al. Expression of somatostatin receptor 2 in Somatotropinoma correlated with the short-term efficacy of somatostatin analogues. International Journal of Endocrinology. 2017;**2017**:9606985. DOI: 10.1155/2017/9606985

[39] Albarel F, Cuny N, Graillon N, Dufour T, et al. Preoperative medical treatment for patients with acromegaly: Yes or No? Journal of the Endocrine Society. 2022;**6**(9):bvac114. DOI: 10.1210/jendso/bvac114

[40] Selek A, Cetinarslan B, Canturk Z, et al. The effect of somatostatin analogues on Ki-67 levels in GH-secreting adenomas. Growth Hormone & IGF Research. 2019;**45**:1-5

[41] Colao A, Auriemma RS, Pivonello R. The effects of somatostatin analogue therapy on pituitary tumor volume in patients with acromegaly. Pituitary. 2016;**19**:210-221. DOI: 10.1007/s11102-015-0677-y

[42] Petersenn S, Houchard A, Sert C, Caron PJ, et al. Predictive factors for

responses to primary medical treatment with lanreotide autogel 120 mg in acromegaly: Post hoc analyses from the PRIMARYS study. Pituitary. 2020;**23**(2):171-181. DOI: 10.1007/s11102-019-01020-3

[43] Colao A, Auriemma RS, Lombardi G, Pivonello R. Resistance to somatostatin analogs in acromegaly. Endocrine Reviews. 2011;**32**:247-271. DOI: 10.1210/er.2010-0002

[44] Kasuki L, Wildemberg LE, Gadelha M. Management of endocrine disease: Personalized medicine in the treatment of acromegaly. European Journal of Endocrinology 2018, Vol. 178, N 3. P. R89-R100. doi: 10.1530/EJE-17-1006

[45] Gadelha MR, Bronstein MD, Brue T, Coculescu M, Freseriu M, Guitelman M, et al. Pasireotide versus continued treatment with octreotide or lanreotide in patients with inadequately controlled acromegaly (PAOLA): A randomised, phase 3 trial. The Lancet Diabetes and Endocrinology. 2014;**2**:875-884. DOI: 10.1016/S2213-8587(14)70169-X

[46] Shimon I, Adnan Z, Gorshtein A, et al. Efficacy and safety of long-acting pasireotide in patients with somatostatin-resistant acromegaly: A multicenter study. Endocrine. 2018;**62**(2):448-455

[47] Coopmans EC, Schneiders JJ, El-Sayed N, Erler NS, Hofland LJ, van der Lely AJ, et al. T2-signal intensity, SSTR expression, and somatostatin analogs efficacy predict response to pasireotide in acromegaly. European Journal of Endocrinology. 2020;**182**(6):595-605. DOI: 10.1530/EJE-19-0840

[48] Stelmachowska-Banas M, Czajka-Oraniec I, Tomasik A, Zgliczynski W. Real-world experience with pasireotide-LAR in resistant acromegaly: A single center 1-year observation. Pituitary. 2022;**25**(1):180-190. DOI: 10.1007/s11102-021-01185-w

[49] Puig-Domingo M, Soto A, Venegas E. Use of lanreotide in combination with cabergoline or pegvisomant in patients with acromegaly in the clinical practice: The ACROCOMB study. Endocrinología y Nutrición. 2016;**63**(8):397-408

[50] Ghajar A, Jones PS, Guarda FJ, Faje A, Tritos NA, Miller KK, et al. Biochemical control in acromegaly with multimodality therapies: Outcomes from a pituitary center and changes over time. The Journal of Clinical Endocrinology and Metabolism. 2020;**105**(3):dgz187. DOI: 10.1210/clinem/dgz187

[51] Fleseriu M, Fuhrer-Sakel D, van der Lely AJ, et al. More than a decade of real-world experience of pegvisomant for acromegaly: ACROSTUDY. European Journal of Endocrinology. 2021;**185**(4):525-538. DOI: 10.1530/EJE-21-0239

[52] Franck SE, Muhammad A, van der Lely AJ, Neggers SJCMM. Combined treatment of somatostatin analogues with pegvisomant in acromegaly. Endocrine. 2016;**52**(2):206-213. DOI: 10.1007/s12020-015-0810-8

[53] Rass L, Rahvar A-H, Matschke J, Satger W, et al. Differences in somatostatin receptor subtype expression in patients with acromegaly: New directions for targeted therapy? Hormones (Athens, Greece) 2022; Vol. 21, N 1. P. 79-89. doi: 10.1007/s42000-021-00327-w

[54] Henriques DG, Lamback EB, Desonne RS, Kasuki L, Gadelha MR. MicroRNA in acromegaly: Involvement in the pathogenesis and in the response to first-generation somatostatin receptor

ligands. International Journal of Molecular Sciences. 2022;**23**(15):8653. DOI: 10.3390/ijms23158653

[55] Störmann S., Schopohl J., Bullmann C., Terkamp C. et al. Multicenter, observational study of Lanreotide autogel for the treatment of patients with acromegaly in routine clinical practice in Germany, Austria and Switzerland. Experimental and Clinical Endocrinology & Diabetes 2021; Vol. 129, N 3. P. 224-233. doi: 10.1055/a-1247-4713

[56] Durmus ET, Atmaca A, Kefeli M, Caliskan S, et al. Age, GH/IGF-1 levels, tumor volume, T2 hypointensity, and tumor subtype rather than proliferation and invasion are all reliable predictors of biochemical response to somatostatin analogue therapy in patients with acromegaly: A clinicopathological study. Growth Hormone & IGF Research. 2022;**67**:101502. DOI: 10.1016/j.ghir.2022.101502

[57] Puig-Domingo M, Bernabéu I, Picó A, Biagetti B, et al. Pasireotide in the personalized treatment of acromegaly. Frontiers in Endocrinology (Lausanne). 2021;**12**:648411. DOI: 10.3389/fendo.2021.648411

[58] Coopmans EC, Korevaar TIM, van Meyel SWF, Daly AF, et al. Multivariable prediction model for biochemical response to first-generation somatostatin receptor ligands in Acromegal. The Journal of Clinics in Endocrinology and Metabolism. 2020;**105**(9):dgaa387. DOI: 10.1210/clinem/dgaa387

[59] Amarawardena W.K.M.G, Liyanarachchi KD, Newell-Price JDC, Ross RJM, et al. Pasireotide: Successful treatment of a sparsely granulated tumour in a resistant case of acromegaly//endocrinology, Diabetes & Metabolism Case Reports. 2017; Vol. 2017, N 1, 17-0067. doi: 10.1530/EDM-17-0067

[60] Kontogeorgos G, Markussis V, Thodou E, Kyrodimou E, et al. Association of Pathology Markers with somatostatin analogue responsiveness in acromegaly. International Journal of Endocrinology. 2022;**2022**:8660470. DOI: 10.1155/2022/8660470

[61] Lim DST, Freseriu M. Personalized medical treatment of patients with acromegaly: A review. Endocrine Practice. 2022;**28**(3):321-332. DOI: 10.1016/j.eprac.2021.12.017

[62] Kasuki L, Wildemberg LE, Neto LV, Marcondes J, et al. Ki-67 is a predictor of acromegaly control with octreotide LAR independent of SSTR2 status and relates to cytokeratin pattern. European Journal of Endocrinology. 2013;**169**(2):217-223. DOI: 10.1530/EJE-13-0349

[63] Gil J, Marques-Pamies M, Sampedro M, Webb SM, et al. Data mining analyses for precision medicine in acromegaly: A proof of concept. Scientific Reports 2022. Vol. 12, N 1. 8979. doi: 10.1038/s41598-022-12955-2

[64] Antsiferov MB, Alekseeva TM, Pronin EV, Pronin VS. Predictors of acromegaly clinical history and treatment effectiveness. (Based on Moscow register data). Endocrinology (News, Opinions, Training). 2020;**10**(3):26-38

[65] Pronin EV, Antsiferov MB, AlekseevaTM, UrusovaLS, LapshinaAM, Mokrysheva NG. Optimization of drug treatment of acromegaly (clinical and morphological comparison). Pharmateca. 2022;**29**(4):44-52. DOI: 10.18565/pharmateca.2022.4.44-52

[66] Ezzat S, Caspar-bell GM, Chik CL, Denis M-C, et al. Predictive markers for postsurgical medical management of acromegaly: A systematic review and consensus treatment guideline. Endocrine Practice. 2019;**25**(4):379-393. DOI: 10.4158/ep-2018-0500

Section 2

Operative Nuances in Pituitary Surgery

Chapter 3

Diaphragma Sellotomy: A Safe Technique to Confirm Adequate Decompression of Optic Chiasm

Vikram Chakravarthy, Vadim Gospodarev, Jorrdan Bissell, Brandon Edelbach, Timothy Marc Eastin and Kenneth De Los Reyes

Abstract

Optic chiasm decompression for preservation of vision is often the primary surgical goal for patients with pituitary tumors. Descent of the diaphragma sellae (DS) is an intraoperative surrogate marker of adequate chiasm decompression. DS may not always descend in an obvious or symmetrical manner, leaving uncertainty to whether the operation was successful. We propose a technique of intentionally incising the DS to ensure adequate chiasm decompression. Here we present patients with pituitary tumors who underwent transsphenoidal surgery and DS incision when the DS was not easily identified and/or did not descend. The approximately 3-mm incision under endoscopic guidance allowed for direct visualization of the suprasellar cistern and optic chiasm. Cerebrospinal fluid (CSF) leak was repaired using a nasoseptal flap in 4 cases, while intradural substitute and thrombin glue were utilized in another case. Five patients with pituitary macroadenomas (average size: 6.4 cm^3) had endoscopic endonasal transsphenoidal resection. Vision improved in all cases postoperatively. There were no postoperative complications or CSF leaks at 1 year. Diaphragma sellotomy ensures chiasm decompression with minimal risk to the patient with current reconstructive techniques and without the need for intraoperative magnetic resonance imaging (iMRI) and reduction of the need for repeated surgical intervention.

Keywords: pituitary, tumor, macroadenoma, neurosurgery, Diaphragma Sella, optic chiasm

1. Introduction

Descent of the diaphragma sellae (DS) during endonasal endoscopic surgery is what surgeons use as a surrogate to determine whether or not enough tumor has been removed to decompress the optic chiasm [1, 2]. The optic chiasm is not directly visible even after removal of the tumor [3]. Ideally, once the tumor is removed, the DS, which is a barrier between the sella and the subarachnoid space, would bow into the field, suggesting successful decompression of the optic chiasm [1, 2]. An ongoing issue in endoscopic transsphenoidal surgery is that the DS is not always identifiable as often times, and the tumor develops a capsule that adheres to the DS, which makes it difficult for the surgeon to differentiate between the two [1–3]. Even when utilizing an endoscope, which allows direct visualization of the sella, multiple intraoperative MRI imaging studies have revealed that there is approximately a 30–66% chance that one may think that they have decompressed the optic chiasm while they have not actually done so [4–9]. Highly successful outcomes associated with utilization of modern techniques of intraoperative cerebrospinal fluid (CSF) leak repair [10–16] allow surgeons to develop innovative approaches to tumor resection, which, in our retrospective study, may ensure decompression of the optic chiasm and reduce the chance of reoperation, without the use of costly intraoperative imaging. In this study, we analyzed the safety and feasibility of a novel technique of "diaphragma sellotomy" to assess, with direct visualization, optic chiasm decompression and extent of tumor removal, without the use of intraoperative imaging. We present a series of five patients with pituitary macroadenomas (average size: 6.4 cm^3) who have undergone endoscopic endonasal transsphenoidal resection. The goal of surgery in each case was chiasm decompression, as each patient suffered rapid and severe vision loss. Successful intraoperative diaphragma sellotomy confirmed chiasm decompression and subsequent CSF leak repair resulted in no postoperative complications. The optic chiasm was directly visualized in all cases. Vision improved in four out of five cases postoperatively, an exception occurred in a patient with a recurrent Rathke's cleft cyst that required multiple resections at other institutions. There were no postoperative CSF leaks at 1 year. This novel technique is a facile and safe way to ensure the goals of surgery have been met with minimal risk.

2. Methods

A retrospective chart review was conducted that analyzed outcomes in patients with pituitary adenomas associated with profound visual deterioration who underwent transsphenoidal surgery and diaphragma sellotomy. The diaphragma sellotomy procedure was performed only when the DS was not easily identified and/or did not descend symmetrically into the field of view. The 3-mm incision allowed for direct visualization of the suprasellar cistern and optic chiasm, which allowed for confirmation of optic chiasm decompression and avoided the need for re-operation. The resultant CSF leaks were repaired using a nasoseptal flap in four cases, and intradural substitute and thrombin glue were utilized in another case. All patients had MRIs and neurological examination of visual fields prior to surgery and at 3 months post-operatively. All patients were neurologically assessed in clinic one-year post surgery.

3. Results

3.1 Demographic and presenting features

After a retrospective chart review of patients undergoing pituitary surgery at our institution, five were selected as having additionally undergone diaphragma sellotomy to assess, with direct visualization, optic chiasm decompression, and extent of tumor removal. Two patients were female and three were male. Their average age at presentation was 48.6 (range 18–69 years). Average body mass index (BMI) was 29.02 kg/m^2 (range 24.7–35.4 kg/m^2). Average size of pituitary macroadenomas was 6.4 cm^3 (range 2.3–13.2 cm^3). All patients initially presented with peripheral field vision loss, which improved in all cases but one, postoperatively. The patient in whom vision did not improve post-operatively had a history of a recurrent Rathke's cleft cyst that required multiple resections at other institutions. There were no postoperative complications or CSF leaks at a 1-year follow-up clinic visit.

3.2 Case illustration

A 69-year-old male with past medical history significant for diabetes mellitus type II presented to our institution's neurosurgery clinic with chief complaints of frontal headaches and peripheral vision loss. The patient first noticed changes in his vision approximately one and half years prior to his visit. He was previously diagnosed with a pituitary tumor *via* magnetic resonance imaging (MRI) at a different institution. However, his vision had progressively worsened over a 3-month period of time, thereby taking a toll on his performance as an avid pickleball player, and eventually led to his presentation at our facility. Neurological exam was unremarkable except upon the assessment of visual fields, and it was determined that the patient had marked left temporal and superior right quadrant visual field deficits. Pre-operative MRI revealed a heterogeneously enhancing sellar/suprasellar mass, which was 2.2 cm anteroposterior x 2.5 cm transverse x 3.2 cm craniocaudal (**Figure 1**) and was therefore determined to be the root cause of significant compression of the patient's optic chiasm. Intraoperatively, the tumor was removed off of the diaphragma sellae and pseudocapsule. Because the diaphragma sellae did not herniate and was not decompressed fully, tuberculum sellae was then further opened using Kerrison rongeurs, and the asymmetrically descended diaphragma sellae was opened from above, superiorly, using the retractable blade in a horizontal fashion (**Figure 2**). Once the supradiaphragmatic space was identified, CSF and the optic chiasm were visualized, and it was confirmed that the optic chiasm had been decompressed (**Figure 3**). After thorough irrigation and hemostasis were achieved, an intradural

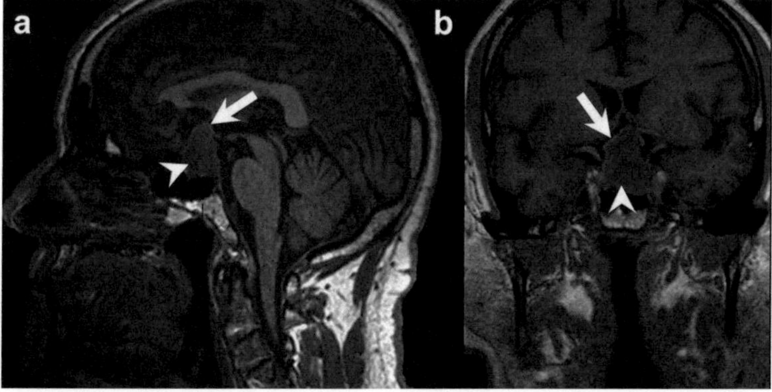

Figure 1.
Pre-operative MRI. A pre-contrast T1 sagittal demonstrating a sellar/suprasellar mass (white arrowhead) isointense to gray matter, compressing the optic chiasm (white arrow). b pre-contrast T1 coronal demonstrating the compressed optic chiasm (white arrow) and mass (white arrowhead).

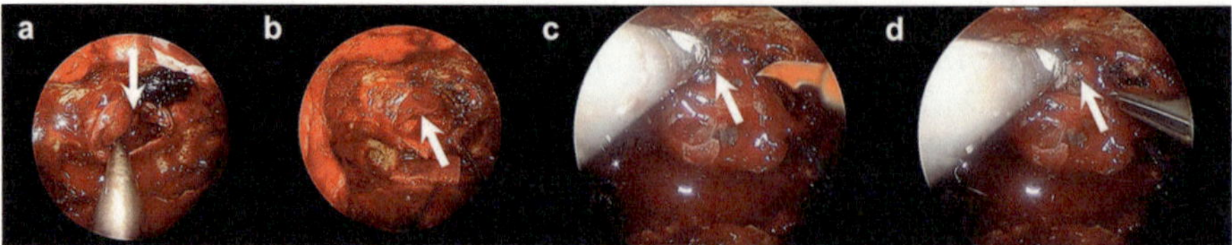

Figure 2.
Intraoperative images of asymmetric descent of DS and incision. A asymmetric descent of DS (white arrow). b residual pituitary gland (white arrow). c incision area (white arrow) in DS. d incision made (white arrow) in DS.

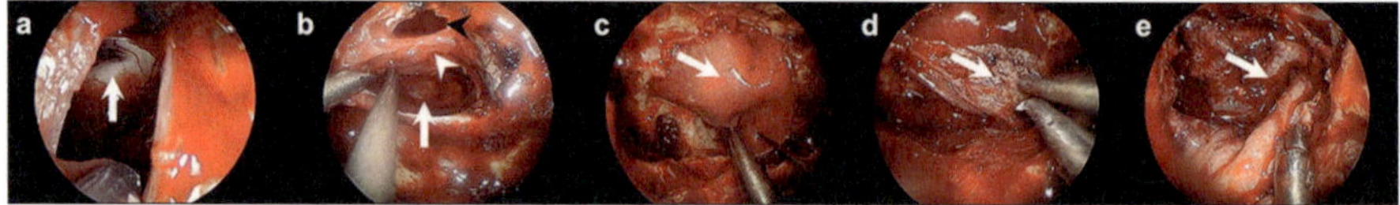

Figure 3.
Intraoperative images of confirmation of decompression and closure. A optic chiasm (white arrow). b Sella (white arrow), diaphragma (white arrowhead), suprasellar space (black arrowhead). c Intradural graft (white arrow). d bone graft across the Sella (white arrow). E Nasoseptal flap (white arrow) covering the defect, no cerebrospinal fluid leak observed.

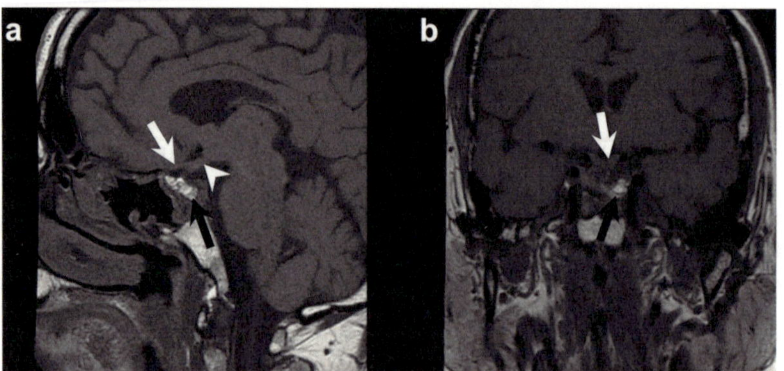

Figure 4.
3-month post-operative MRI. A pre-contrast T1 sagittal demonstrating near total resection of tumor, with optic nerve (white arrow), pituitary stalk (white arrowhead) and fat (black arrow). b pre-contrast T1 coronal demonstrating the decompressed optic chiasm (white arrow) and fat (black arrow).

graft along with a bone graft and a nasoseptal flap were cut and fashioned to be placed in order to cover the defect (**Figure 3**). Surgicel™, Duraseal™, and Gelfoam™ were then placed on top to finalize the closure and observe for a possible CSF leak, the latter of which never occurred. Immediately after surgery the patient noticed improvement in his left visual field. A 3-month post-operative MRI demonstrated near total resection of the pituitary tumor along with a fully decompressed optic chiasm (**Figure 4**). At the 3-month post-operative clinic visit, the patient stated that his vision continued to improve, and he was eager to share that he had finally resumed playing pickleball. Upon neurological exam, the patient's visual fields were fully intact.

4. Discussion

Records of pituitary tumor surgery go back to the early 1900s when common surgical techniques included palliative craniectomies, subfrontal, or subtemporal craniotomies, as well as transnasal transethmoidal, sublabial endonasal-transseptal, and transsphenoidal methods. Unfortunately, mortality rate ranged from 66 to 21%, which was associated with palliative craniectomy and transsphenoidal approach, respectively [17]. However, between 1910 and 1925, Cushing focused exclusively on the transsphenoidal approach which he utilized in 231 pituitary tumor cases and was able to achieve a mortality rate of only 5.6%. It is indubitable that the advent of endoscope allowed for greater visualization of neuroanatomical structures, especially during transsphenoidal surgery, and in addition to modern understanding of microbiology, as well as utilization of aseptic surgical technique, the surgical mortality rate for this procedure is now approximately 0.6% [18].

The decompression and preservation or restoration of vision is often the primary surgical goal in the treatment of patients harboring pituitary macroadenomas with severe optic chiasm compression with up to 80.9% of patients experiencing postoperative improvement in their vision [19]. Despite the success of transsphenoidal surgery overall at improving vision, this success is still dependent on several factors that can be improved upon, including surgical technique. Descent of the diaphragma sellae (DS), a thin, tenuous structure that forms the roof of the sella turcica and covers the pituitary gland, during endonasal endoscopic transsphenoidal surgery is the surrogate marker of adequate chiasm decompression [1–3, 20]. In management of large pituitary lesions, this structure is often difficult to identify, or may be violated by the tumor. At times, it may not descend symmetrically, leaving the surgeon unsure whether the goals of surgery have been met. Due to the difficulty of distinguishing normal pituitary gland, tumor, tumor capsule, and the diaphragma sella, intraoperative MRI (iMRI) has become an increasingly utilized, though cost-prohibitive tool in pituitary surgery, without which the surgeon is able to predict extent of resection in only 65% of cases [21]. Furthermore, the surgeon is often left to finish surgery questioning whether the optic chiasm is decompressed and hoping for future spontaneous diaphragma descent and chiasm decompression if adequate tumor debulking was performed. Our proposed technique of intentionally incising the presumed diaphragma sella allows for assurance of adequate chiasm decompression at the time of surgery. Intraoperatively, the presumed diaphragma sella can be incised to visualize into the subarachnoid space and suprasellar cistern and confirm the extent of optic chiasm decompression. The small low flow CSF leak can be repaired with a number of techniques at the disposal of the skull base surgeon. It is common neurosurgical practice to utilize abdominal fat grafting when a large cavity is encountered after tumor resection to fill the "dead space," as well as a Durepair™ inlay, Duraseal™, and Surgicel™ [22–24]. Nasoseptal flaps are typically reserved only for large, high flow CSF leaks [25]. Current trends in pituitary surgery advocate against intentional opening of the diaphragma sella, as this increases the risk of a postoperative CSF leak. More recent studies have shown that despite intraoperative CSF leak, with proper reconstruction techniques, postoperative CSF leak rates are exceedingly low and range from 0.6 to 2.3% and can be easily managed or even completely prevented with utilization of lumbar drainage [11, 24, 26]. With the main goal of vision preservation and restoration, diaphragma sellotomy ensures the goals of surgery are met with minimal risk to the patient, while also allowing for pituitary gland preservation; repeat surgery stemming from patients reporting marginal clinical improvement along with radiographic studies demonstrating persistent optic chiasm compression, can be avoided.

5. Conclusion

Optic chiasm decompression is often the primary surgical goal for patients with pituitary macroadenomas. Descent of the diaphragma sellae (DS) indicates chiasm decompression. DS is not always identifiable and its descent not always symmetric. Intraoperative MRI (iMRI) has become an increasingly utilized, though cost-prohibitive tool to confirm decompression. Diaphragma sellotomy ensures chiasm decompression with minimal risk to the patient with current reconstructive techniques and without the need for iMRI. Repeat immediate or delayed surgery to ensure chiasm decompression can be avoided. Diaphragma sellotomy is a facile and safe way to ensure the goals of surgery have been met with minimal risk. Utilization of this novel technique may allow for more rapid recovery of vision and prevention of repeated surgical intervention.

Compliance with ethical standards

Conflict of interest

The authors declare that they have no conflicts of interest.

Informed consent

Informed consent was not required from participants included in the study. All of the procedural outcomes and test results analyzed were previously collected as part of the course of routine treatment, and no additional interventions were required, thereby waiving the need for informed consent. The authors' institutional review board (IRB) approved waiver of informed consent/authorization for the study.

Ethical approval

All procedures performed in studies involving human participants were in accordance with the ethical standards of the institutional and/or national research committee and with the 1964 Helsinki declaration and its later amendments or comparable ethical standards.

Author details

Vikram Chakravarthy[1], Vadim Gospodarev[2*], Jorrdan Bissell[3], Brandon Edelbach[3], Timothy Marc Eastin[3] and Kenneth De Los Reyes[2]

1 Department of Neurosurgery, Cleveland Clinic Foundation, Cleveland, OH, United States

2 Department of Neurosurgery, Loma Linda University Medical Center, Loma Linda, CA, United States

3 Loma Linda University School of Medicine, Loma Linda, CA, United States

*Address all correspondence to: vgospodarev@llu.edu

References

[1] Guinto Balanzar G, Abdo M, Mercado M, Guinto P, Nishimura E, Arechiga N. Diaphragma sellae: A surgical reference for transsphenoidal resection of pituitary macroadenomas. World Neurosurgery. 2011;**75**:286-293

[2] Honegger J, Ernemann U, Psaras T, Will B. Objective criteria for successful transsphenoidal removal of suprasellar nonfunctioning pituitary adenomas. A prospective study. Acta Neurochirurgica. 2006;**149**:21-29

[3] Rhoton AL. Anatomy of the Pituitary Gland and Sellar Region, in Diagnosis and Management of Pituitary Tumors. Totowa, NJ: Humana Press; 2001. pp. 13-40. Available from: https://link.springer.com/chapter/10.1007/978-1-59259-217-3_2 [Accessed: 16 June 2018]

[4] Berkmann S, Fandino J, Zosso S, Killer HE, Remonda L, Landolt H. Intraoperative magnetic resonance imaging and early prognosis for vision after transsphenoidal surgery for sellar lesions. Journal of Neurosurgery. 2011;**115**:518-527

[5] Boellis A, Espagnet MCR, Romano A, Trillò G, Raco A, Moraschi M, et al. Dynamic intraoperative MRI in transsphenoidal resection of pituitary macroadenomas: A quantitative analysis. Journal of Magnetic Resonance Imaging. 2014;**40**:668-673

[6] Bohinski RJ, Warnick RE, Gaskill-Shipley MF, Zuccarello M, van Loveren HR, Kormos DW, et al. Intraoperative magnetic resonance imaging to determine the extent of resection of pituitary macroadenomas during transsphenoidal microsurgery. Neurosurgery. 2001;**49**:1133-1143; discussion 1143-1144,

[7] Szerlip NJ, Zhang Y-C, PlacantonakisDG,GoldmanM,ColevasKB, Rubin DG, et al. Transsphenoidal resection of Sellar Tumors using high-field intraoperative magnetic resonance imaging. Skull Base. 2011;**21**:223-232

[8] Vitaz TW, Inkabi KE, Carrubba CJ. Intraoperative MRI for transphenoidal procedures: Short-term outcome for 100 consecutive cases. Clinical Neurology and Neurosurgery. 2011;**113**:731-735

[9] Walker DG, Black PM. Use of intraoperative MRI in pituitary surgery. Operative Techniques in Neurosurgery. 2002;**5**:231-238

[10] Burkett CJ, Patel S, Tabor MH, Padhya T, Vale FL. Polyethylene glycol (PEG) hydrogel dural sealant and collagen dural graft matrix in transsphenoidal pituitary surgery for prevention of postoperative cerebrospinal fluid leaks. Journal of Clinical Neuroscience. 2011;**18**:1513-1517

[11] Cappabianca P, Cavallo LM, Esposito F, Valente V, de Divitiis E. Sellar repair in endoscopic Endonasal Transsphenoidal surgery: Results of 170 cases. Neurosurgery. 2002;**51**:1365-1372

[12] Kaptain GJ, Kanter AS, Hamilton DK, Laws ER. Management and implications of intraoperative cerebrospinal fluid leak in transnasoseptal transsphenoidal microsurgery. Neurosurgery. 2011;**68**(1 Suppl Operative):144-151

[13] Locatelli D, Vitali M, Custodi VM, Scagnelli P, Castelnuovo P, Canevari FR. Endonasal approaches to the sellar and parasellar regions: Closure

techniques using biomaterials. Acta Neurochirurgica. 2009;**151**:1431-1437

[14] Nishioka H, Izawa H, Ikeda Y, Namatame H, Fukami S, Haraoka J. Dural suturing for repair of cerebrospinal fluid leak in transnasal transsphenoidal surgery. Acta Neurochirurgica. 2009;**151**:1427-1430

[15] Sade B, Mohr G, Frenkiel S. Management of intra-operative cerebrospinal fluid leak in transnasal transsphenoidal pituitary microsurgery: Use of post-operative lumbar drain and sellar reconstruction without fat packing. Acta Neurochirurgica. 2005;**148**:13-19

[16] Seiler RW, Mariani L. Sellar reconstruction with resorbable vicryl patches, gelatin foam, and fibrin glue in transsphenoidal surgery: A 10-year experience with 376 patients. Journal of Neurosurgery. 2000;**93**:762-765

[17] Pascual JM, Mongardi L, Prieto R, Castro-Dufourny I, Rosdolsky M, Strauss S, et al. Giovanni Verga (1879-1923), author of a pioneering treatise on pituitary surgery: The foundations of this new field in Europe in the early 1900s. Neurosurgical Review. 2017;**40**:559-575

[18] Halvorsen H, Ramm-Pettersen J, Josefsen R, Rønning P, Reinlie S, Meling T, et al. Surgical complications after transsphenoidal microscopic and endoscopic surgery for pituitary adenoma: A consecutive series of 506 procedures. Acta Neurochirurgica. 2014;**156**:441-449

[19] Muskens IS, Zamanipoor Najafabadi AH, Briceno V, Lamba N, Senders JT, van Furth WR, et al. Visual outcomes after endoscopic endonasal pituitary adenoma resection: A systematic review and meta-analysis. Pituitary. 2017;**20**:539-552

[20] Renn WH, Rhoton AL. Microsurgical anatomy of the sellar region. Journal of Neurosurgery. 1975;**43**:288-298

[21] Zaidi HA, De Los RK, Barkhoudarian G, Litvack ZN, Bi WL, Rincon-Torroella J, et al. The utility of high-resolution intraoperative MRI in endoscopic transsphenoidal surgery for pituitary macroadenomas: Early experience in the advanced multimodality image guided operating suite. Neurosurgical Focus. 2016;**40**:E18

[22] Gondim JA, Schops M, de Almeida JPC, de Albuquerque LAF, Gomes E, Ferraz T, et al. Endoscopic endonasal transsphenoidal surgery: Surgical results of 228 pituitary adenomas treated in a pituitary center. Pituitary. 2009;**13**:68-77

[23] Hofstetter CP, Shin BJ, Mubita L, Huang C, Anand VK, Boockvar JA, et al. Endoscopic endonasal transsphenoidal surgery for functional pituitary adenomas. Neurosurgical Focus. 2011;**30**:E10

[24] Wang F, Zhou T, Wei S, Meng X, Zhang J, Hou Y, et al. Endoscopic endonasal transsphenoidal surgery of 1,166 pituitary adenomas. Surgical Endoscopy. 2015;**29**:1270-1280

[25] Liu JK, Schmidt RF, Choudhry OJ, Shukla PA, Eloy JA. Surgical nuances for nasoseptal flap reconstruction of cranial base defects with high-flow cerebrospinal fluid leaks after endoscopic skull base surgery. Neurosurgical Focus. 2012;**32**:E7

[26] Tamasauskas A, Sinkūnas K, Draf W, Deltuva V, Matukevicius A, Rastenyte D, et al. Management of cerebrospinal fluid leak after surgical removal of pituitary adenomas. Medicina Kaunas Lithuania. 2008;**44**:302-307

Section 3

Role of Pituitary Gland in Reproductive Medicine

Chapter 4

Role of Pituitary Gland in Fertility Preservation

Eniola Risikat Kadir, Abdulmalik Omogbolahan Hussein, Lekan Sheriff Ojulari and Gabriel O. Omotoso

Abstract

The pituitary gland is one of the major organs that make up the endocrine system. The pituitary gland secretes various hormones some of which acts on target organs specifically and some that act on other endocrine bodies to stimulate or inhibit production of hormones based on response to different signals in the body. The pituitary gland is also regulated by hormones released from the hypothalamus and hence, the hypothalamus and pituitary gland coalesce to form a central control unit for endocrine processes throughout the body. Of its numerous functions, the pituitary is very vital in reproduction as it regulates hormones that are necessary for reproductive functions in the body. This chapter discusses at length, the importance and role of the pituitary gland in reproduction. Basically, the pituitary gland responds to stimuli from the hypothalamus to produce hormones that act on the gonads (testes and ovaries) to produce sex hormones that are necessary for sexual maturation. The hypothalamus, pituitary gland and the gonads form a network for the communication via the hypothalamo-pituitary-gonadal axis and it allows efficiency in stimulating and inhibiting release of hormones via a feedback mechanism. The optimum functioning of the pituitary gland is absolutely necessary to facilitate a healthy reproductive functioning and avoid reproductive complications like infertility. Conception should be a natural part of life that should occur spontaneously and approximately 15–25% of couples within the reproductive age are struggling to conceive, and require medical attention to achieve this and only about 1–2% of couples are sterile. Infertility cases that result from pituitary gland-related complications can be caused by a number of factors either congenital or acquired. Recent research inferences on the pathophysiology of infertility have identified the overproduction of reactive oxygen species as an important factor in infertility. There are various studies regarding the effects of endocrine-disrupting chemicals (an environmental pollutant) on the reproductive functions of animals which can be through alterations in a hormonal milieu as well as reactive oxygen species. It therefore becomes imperative to look into effects of the environment on the endocrine pathways and its reflection on fertility. This chapter also looked into some of the causative factors of these disorders and the risk the pose to a reproductive health.

Keywords: pituitary gland, fertility, bisphenol-A, endocrine system, reproductive health

1. Introduction

The pituitary gland is a miniature endocrine organ that is situated at the base of the brain directly underneath the hypothalamus. It is suspended from the base of the brain by the infundibulum which is otherwise known as the pituitary stalk and it is situated within a small groove on the sphenoid bone. The pituitary gland is structurally and functionally considered as a double structure because it has 2 distinct parts—the anterior pituitary (adenohypophysis) and the posterior pituitary (neurohypophysis) which are of different embryonic origin and are specific in their own respective functions. The pituitary is sometimes referred to as the "master gland" because other than secreting its own hormones, it also controls secretion of hormones by other endocrine organs as responses to different signals in the body. The pituitary is capable of controlling all these other endocrine processes by forming a hypothalamo-pituitary complex which functions as central control for the brain to organize important processes in the body. The hypothalamo-pituitary complex controls these processes forming a circuit with target endocrine organs, these circuit is known as axis. This axis forms a kind of feedback loop which helps to stimulate or inhibit release of hormones from the hypothalamus and pituitary alike. The importance of the pituitary gland can be inferred by understanding the numerous functions that it serves in the body. Some of the functions of the pituitary gland include; regulation of body metabolism, growth and development, homeostasis and also reproduction. The pituitary is capable of exhibiting all of the aforementioned functions by actions of different hormones that it releases to different target organs in the body. Some of the hormones produced by the pituitary gland include growth hormone, thyroid-stimulating hormone, luteinizing hormone, follicle stimulating hormone, prolactin, oxytocin, etc. For the context of this chapter, there will be an emphasis on its importance in reproduction and fertility. The pituitary acts on the ovaries and testes through the hypothalamo-pituitary-gonadal axis and it controls the reproductive function in females and males through the actions of two hormones—luteinizing hormone and follicle stimulating hormone. In immediate pre-pubertal life, production of luteinizing hormone (LH) is usually in low quantities but as puberty begins to set in, LH production increases. This upsurge would cause the stimulation of gonadal steroidogenesis which is necessary for sexual maturation. In females, release of LH and follicle-stimulating hormone (FSH) which is triggered by the secretion of gonadotropin releasing hormone (GnRH), otherwise called luteinizing hormone releasing hormone (LHRH) from the hypothalamus helps to regulate the reproductive system. Once secreted, the LH and FSH act on the ovaries to stimulate ovulation and secretion of sex hormones which are estrogen and progesterone. Ovulation is made possible by summative action of the pituitary gland, the hypothalamus and the ovaries. As described earlier, the process kick starts in the hypothalamus which releases hormones that act on the pituitary gland to release gonadotropins (LH and FSH) which then acts directly on the ovaries. In the ovarian follicles, there are 3 types of cells; the theca, the granulosa and the oocyte. LH acts on the theca cells to produce androstenedione, FSH then stimulates aromatase to act on the androstenedione to produce estradiol. Once estradiol is produced, it causes a positive feedback on LH release by blocking off negative feedback that is caused by estrogen. The further release of LH would then cause an "LH surge," which would in turn initiate the ovulation process. After the event of ovulation, the ovarian follicle turns into the corpus luteum. The corpus luteum is responsible for secretion of progesterone and human chorionic gonadotropin in the event of a pregnancy. In males, the release of FSH and LH by the pituitary gland is responsible for spermatogenesis—production of sperm and the secretion of testosterone, the male sex hormone.

2. Factors that can affect normal functioning of the pituitary gland

It is important that there is a balance in the level of hormones that is being produced by the pituitary gland to allow proper functioning of the reproductive systems. Hormonal imbalances resulting from incompetence of the pituitary gland can have huge ramifications on the reproductive systems and ultimately resulting in fertility complications. Several factors can be held responsible for improper functioning of the pituitary gland, some of these factors are;

- Tumors: Pituitary tumors (also known as pituitary adenomas) are slow-growing non-cancerous growths on the pituitary gland. These tumors are categorized into two; non-functioning adenomas (or non-secreting) and functioning adenomas (or secreting). The non-functioning adenomas do not secrete any hormones but can grow uncontrollably large which might require surgical removal and in rare cases, the tumor can rupture and result in internal hemorrhage. The functioning adenomas usually secrete hormones which can directly cause hormonal imbalances that would result in infertility. The functioning adenomas are classified based on the hormones they secrete. A very common type of a functioning adenoma is the prolactinoma, which causes excess release of prolactin. It is responsible for about 40% of all the pituitary tumors and its occurrence is more prevalent in the female populace [1] and also about 15% of total intracranial tumors [2]. Excess production of prolactin (hyperprolactinemia) can cause a range of complications in the reproductive system. Excess prolactin suppresses the action of FSH and LH which causes irregularities in the menstrual cycle and also interferes with ovulation in women and cause inability to conceive in women. It can also cause a condition known as "galactorrhea" which means production of breast milk in women who are not breastfeeding or even pregnant. In men, suppressed action of FSH and LH can impede spermatogenesis and cause impotence. It can also cause low sex drive in both sexes.

- Trauma: Physical infarctions to the pituitary gland resulting from head injuries such as skull fractures or concussions can damage the gland and stop its functioning which would result in hormonal imbalances which in turn translates to infertility. Some other symptoms that might result from trauma to the pituitary gland include fatigue, headaches and vision problems.

- Auto-immune diseases: Diseases like hypophysitis where the body defenses attack the pituitary gland and cause inflammation and damage to the gland. This can also lead to hormonal imbalances and cause fertility problems.

- Infections: Some infections like meningitis and tuberculosis can affect the functioning of the pituitary gland. The causative bacteria of tuberculosis "mycobacterium tuberculosis" which majorly infects the lungs is also capable of affecting other parts of the body including the pituitary gland. Its malfunctioning can result when the bacteria affects the pituitary gland, a condition called tuberculous hypophysitis of the pituitary gland.

- Medications such as antidepressants, antipsychotics and chemotherapy drugs can affect the normal functioning of the pituitary gland and cause hormonal imbalances.

- Radiation therapy: Radiation exposure to the skull for treatment of intracranial malignancies alter the proper functioning of the pituitary gland.

All the aforementioned factors can affect the pituitary gland and lead to hormonal imbalances by either causing over activity or under activity of the gland. These conditions are known as hyperpituitarism and hypopituitarism respectively.

3. Effects of pituitary gland dysfunction on reproduction and fertility

3.1 Hyperpituitarism

Hyperpituitarism, a condition where there is excessive secretion of pituitary hormones can be largely associated with functional pituitary adenomas which can stimulate excess hormone secretion (e.g. prolactinoma). The complications that result from this however depends on the particular hormone that is being over secreted. The most commonly affected hormones in hyperpituitarism are growth hormone and prolactin. Although both hormones are not directly involved with fertility, prolactin is an important hormone for secondary sexual characters which includes breast development and production of milk in pregnant and lactating mothers. Also, excess prolactin can suppress the production of estrogen and testosterone which influences fertility by causing anovulation in females and decreased sperm production and quality in males. Hyperpituitarism is mostly treated using medication regimen, however the approach to managing the condition may depend on the cause and severity. Other ways of managing hyperpituitarism are the surgical approach and radiotherapy.

3.2 Hypopituitarism

Hypopituitarism is a condition where the pituitary gland cannot produce hormones in the required amounts for proper functioning. Hypopituitarism is the absolute or partial loss of the pituitary gland (anterior and posterior) function that can result from hypothalamic or pituitary disorders [3]. It is less prevalent in comparison to hyperpituitarism. Also, some other contributing factors like the cause of the hypopituitarism, the age of onset and the severity of the hormone deficiency can affect the clinical presentation of the clinical state. Depending on the etiology of the hypopituitarism, the condition can be categorized into two groups—primary and secondary hypopituitarism.

3.2.1 Primary hypopituitarism

In primary hypopituitarism, the condition is caused by disorders of the pituitary gland which can be caused by damage or inadequate functioning of the pituitary hormone secreting cells. Other causes of this condition are tumors (pituitary adenomas), surgical complications and exposure to radiation in therapy. In cases related with adenomas, the onset of the condition is usually slow. However, in patients who suffer from pituitary hemorrhage or lack of blood supply to the pituitary gland, a medical condition referred to as pituitary apoplexy, the onset of the hypopituitarism is normally quick and symptoms may begin to prevail within hours. This is as seen in postpartum hemorrhage or in trauma where the blood loss is massive and replacement wasn't commensurate with the loss.

3.2.2 Secondary hypopituitarism

In secondary hypopituitarism, the condition is associated with complication with the hypothalamus. This could be from damage to the infundibulum (pituitary stalk) which is often caused by trauma to the head or neck. Also tumor growth in proximity of the *sella turcica* if big enough, can exert pressure on the pituitary stalk and cause a lesion. In surgical attempts to remove such types of tumor (sellar or parasellar tumors), the pituitary stalk is highly exposed and is at a great risk of being damaged and this can lead to secondary hypopituitarism.

Like hyperpituitarism, the clinical presentation largely depends on the specific pituitary hormone that is being under-produced. In regards to reproduction and fertility, the gonadotropins are the major hormones of concern. However, symptoms and clinical presentation of low gonadotropins depends on the stage of onset (pre-pubertal or post puberty). Some of the symptoms are listed below;

- Exaggerated decrease in size of penis and absence of testicles.
- Lack of development of secondary sexual features during puberty (e.g. breasts and pubic hair).
- Low sex drive and desire in adulthood.
- Fertility complications in adulthood.

3.3 Pituitary hyperplasia

This is associated with a rapid increase in the number of one or more cell subtypes of the pituitary gland. These increments are characterized by an enlargement of the pituitary gland. It can occur as a result of physiological or pathological changes in the body. Pregnancy state is a period where there are numerous physiological changes in the body. During pregnancy, the pituitary gland increases in weight and size by almost one-third of its original size. This inflammation is caused by activation of lactotroph cells which in turn causes stimulation of prolactin [4]. Prolactin stimulation helps preparing the mother for lactation and breastfeeding. Although, the condition is reversible in the normal physiological conditions like pregnancy, other inflammations resulting from pathological effects may require medical intervention for their management.

4. The hypothalamo-pituitary gonadal axis and its role in reproduction

The hypothalamo-pituitary-gonadal axis (HPG axis) is a complex system that is in charge of controlling and regulation of hormones that are persistent with reproductive function and fertility in both males and females. As stated earlier, a typical hypothalamo-pituitary axis consists of the hypothalamus, the pituitary gland and the target organs terminally. The target organs of the HPG axis are the gonads, which are specifically the ovaries and testes in males and females respectively. The first component, the hypothalamus, is a small organ that is located deep within the center of the brain and directly above the pituitary gland—the pituitary gland is suspended from the hypothalamus by the pituitary stalk. The hypothalamus is a vital organ for regulating numerous physiological functions in the body one of which is the regulation of release of pituitary hormones. However, the hypothalamus is also capable of secreting its own hormones, the hormones released by the hypothalamus are widely categorized into two; tropic hormones which are hormones that act directly on different target organs in the body, and hypophysiotropic hormones which are released to act on the pituitary gland. The hypothalamus is largely connected with different parts of the central nervous system (CNS) but it is however most closely related and connected to the pituitary gland due to their interwoven actions and their close proximity to each other. This tightly connected formation gives rise to the hypothalamo-pituitary complex. This complex then forms an axis by terminally connecting to different target organs. These axes include hypothalamo-pituitary gonadal (HPG) axis, hypothalamo-pituitary-adrenal axis, hypothalamo-pituitary-thyroid axis and also the growth hormone axis. The HPG axis serves a variety of functions in the body which includes development of the immune system, aging but most importantly reproduction. The mechanism of action of the HPG axis begins at the hypothalamus by releasing gonadotropin-releasing hormones (GnRH) which is an example of hypophysiotropic hormone because it acts directly on the pituitary gland to release gonadotropins. The released gonadotropins (LH and FSH) then acts on the gonads (testes and ovaries) in their own distinct ways which has been explained earlier in this chapter. The HPG axis has distinct actions in both males and females and are also regulated differently by their own respective negative feedback mechanisms which regulates the stimulation and inhibition of release of hormones by the hypothalamus and pituitary gland (**Figure 1**).

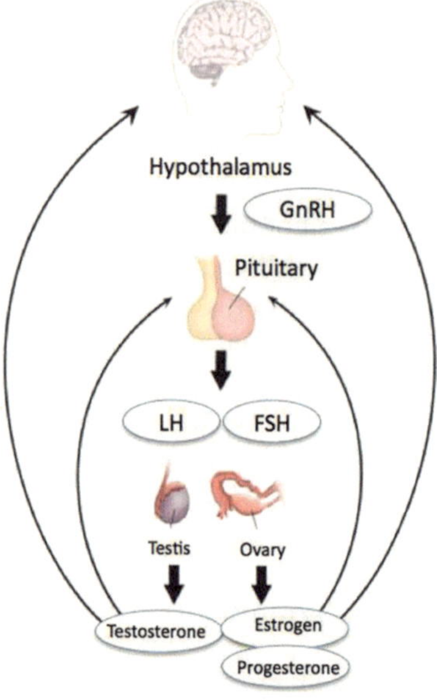

Figure 1.
Diagram showing the dynamic of the hypothalamo-pituitary-gonadal axis [5].

In males, the production of the male sex hormone (testosterone) and also the male gamete (sperm cells) are the primary responsibility of the HPG axis. Production of testosterone is achieved by the bonding of luteinizing hormone (LH) to the interstitial cells of the testes and stimulating the Leydig cells to synthesize it [6]. Spermatogenesis, on the other hand, is stimulated by the follicle-stimulating hormone (FSH). FSH stimulates Sertoli cells which are present in the seminiferous epithelium. The stimulated cells produce a protein complex called the androgen-binding protein (ABP). The ABP synergizes with the already-produced testosterone to provide regulatory molecules and nutrient materials required for maintaining spermatogenesis. Therefore, both the FSH directly and LH indirectly regulate spermatogenesis through the bonding of ABP to testosterone. The HPG axis in males is regulated by a negative feedback effect on the hypothalamus by inhibiting the release of GnRH which in turn halts the release of FSH and LH. The negative feedback is achieved by the release of inhibin by the Sertoli cells which inhibits another protein activin that stimulates the release of gonadotropins by the pituitary gland and hereby indirectly inhibiting the hypothalamus (**Figure 2**).

In females, the HPG axis is primarily concerned with the regulation of the ovarian cycle and the menstrual cycle. As the gonadotropins are released by the pituitary gland, they stimulate the production of estrogen and inhibin by the ovary. Like testosterone in males, estrogen directly inhibits the release of GnRH by the hypothalamus through a negative feedback mechanism. Inhibin here also suppresses activin which indirectly inhibits the hypothalamic release of GnRH. In the reproductive cycle, the development of the ovarian follicle is achieved by a positive feedback loop that involves LH and estrogen. Once the developed follicle releases its ova, there is stimulation of the ovary to produce progesterone. Production of progesterone provides a negative feedback effect that counters the positive feedback of LH and estrogen, and this feedback suppresses the production of GnRH by the hypothalamus which in turn inhibits the release of gonadotropins from the pituitary. In the other

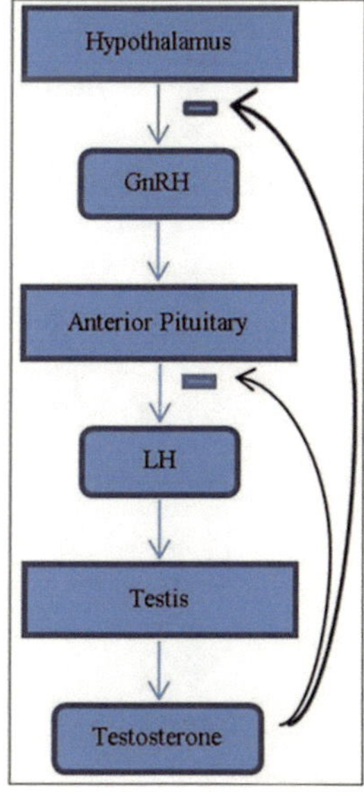

Figure 2.
Diagram showing the feedback loop of the hypothalamo-pituitary-gonadal axis in males [7].

event that the follicle is not fertilized and the onset of menstruation begins, the level of progesterone diminishes and the negative feedback is also overturned which now allows the production of GnRH from the hypothalamus and also the release of the gonadotropins from the pituitary. The released gonadotropins now begin to prepare the next ovarian follicle for the reproductive cycle. The HPG axis is also responsible in the menstrual cycle as the hormones produced by the pituitary are involved in the three phases of the menstrual cycle (**Figure 3**).

The HPG axis is a somewhat complex system that ensures the regulation of hormones that control reproductive functions and fertility. Being an essential benchmark in the endocrine system, its proper functioning is important for reproductive competence and fertility. The HPG axis is closely controlled by various feedback mechanisms that ensure hormones are produced in adequate quantities and at the right time. Any disruption in the normal functioning of the HPG axis is tantamount to having significant ramifications for the reproductive system and fertility which can culminate in reproductive disturbances.

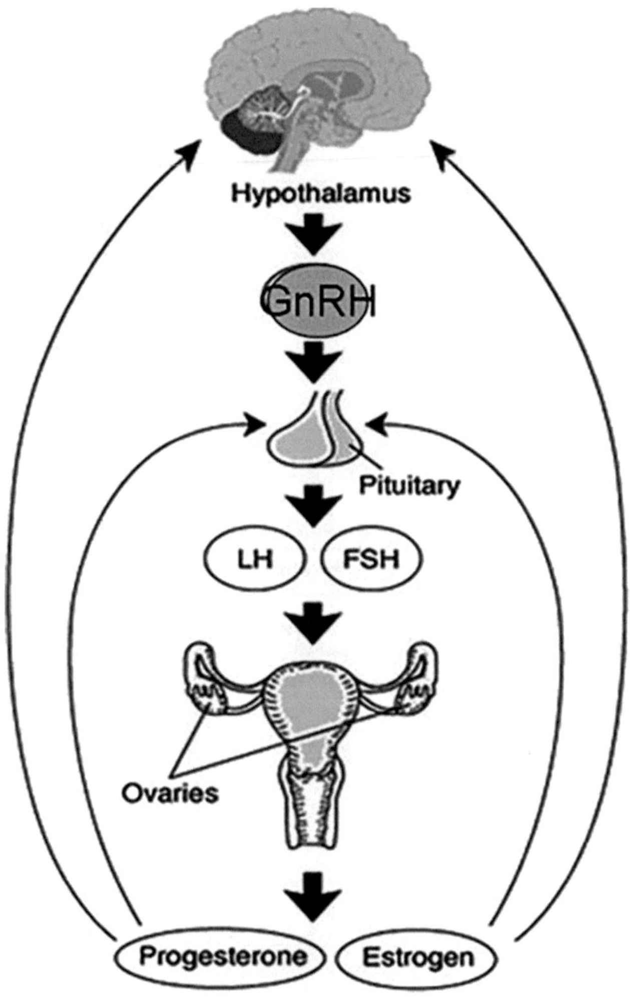

Figure 3.
Diagram showing the feedback loop of the hypothalamo-pituitary-gonadal axis in females [8].

4.1 Disorders of the hypothalamo-pituitary-gonadal axis and their implications on reproduction and fertility

The HPG axis can be affected at any level of its organization (i.e. it can occur at the hypothalamus, pituitary gland and also at the gonads in both sexes), and this can translate to different implications. Although the cause of some of these disorders are generally considered idiopathic, some contributory factors include:

- Genetics: Some of the disorders of the HPG axis are as a result of genetic abnormalities. HPG axis disorders like Klinefelter and Turner syndrome in males and females respectively are as a result of genetic aberrations on the chromosomes.

- Trauma: An injury or physical lesions to the brain or the gonads can disrupt the normal functioning of the HPG axis and can ultimately lead to hormonal imbalances.

- Autoimmune diseases: Such diseases affecting the immune system can affect the ovaries and testes causing interference with the axis thereby causing imbalances.

- Tumors: Abnormal growth(s) can disrupt by stimulating or inhibiting production of hormones.

- Medications: Drugs such as chemotherapy can disrupt hormone production and lead to HPG disorders.

- Environment: Exposure to some environmental elements like chemicals and radiation can interfere with the HPG axis and cause hormonal imbalances. Also environmental toxins like Bisphenol-A (BPA) which is an established endocrine disruptor can directly cause hormonal alterations which can lead to HPG axis disorders.

Some of the disorders that can result from the disruption of the HPG axis include hypogonadism which is a condition whereby the gonads produce little or no sex hormones which will lead to a range of symptoms that are all associated with infertility. Prepubertal affectations can lead to precocious puberty, a condition where there is an abnormal haste or delay in the onset of puberty in the adolescents. Kallmans syndrome is also a genetic disorder which causes failure of puberty due to lack of production of gonadotropin-releasing hormone in the hypothalamus. However, there are more sex-specific disorders that can be caused by the disruption of the HPG axis.

4.2 Effect of environmental toxins (endocrine disruptors) on the pituitary gland and fertility

Over the past decade, studies on the effects of Endocrine Disrupting Chemicals (EDCs) on the reproductive functions of animals have raised some health concerns. In response to these concerns, the World Health Organization (WHO) has several publications, including the recent state of the science of endocrine disrupting chemicals in 2012 [9]. Worldwide, urbanization is progressing with increased demands and use of BPA. It is currently being used in many of our day to day materials such as foods packages, papers, electronics, medical equipments, etc. Therefore, there will be an upsurge in the possible health risks associated with endocrine disrupting chemical exposures. One of such EDC is Bisphenol-A (BPA).

Bisphenol-A is a synthetic chemical that is used in the manufacturing and production of polycarbonates and epoxy resins [10]. These (polycarbonates and epoxy resins) are two types of thermosetting plastics that are widely used in various applications like production of some day-to-day materials for human usage. Some of these materials include; food containers, water bottles, eyeglass lenses and in electronics. Hence, BPA is a very popular chemical compound in our environment. In recent times, a high number of chemicals with endocrine-disrupting abilities have been recorded and they are generally referred to as endocrine-disrupting chemicals (EDCs) [11]. EDCs are exogenous substances that are able to simulate or interfere with the endocrine system hereby remodifying important biological processes like organ development, reproduction, metabolism, etc. [12]. BPA is one of the most common EDCs and it can mimic the action of estrogen and can cause alterations in the endocrine systems which can cause adverse effects on the human reproductive health [13, 14].

Laboratory studies have shown that fetal and neonatal exposure to relatively low doses of BPA may result in reproductive and developmental disorders, including impaired sexual differentiation in the brain [15]. The accumulation of BPA deposits also has clinical implications on the reproductive system since exposure to its low doses during prenatal life has been shown to affect spermatogenesis in the offspring of male rodents. Sex specific changes in the function of infant's hypothalamo-pituitary-adrenal axis, which may culminate in anxiety or depression-like behaviors in offspring, can be associated with prenatal exposure to BPA [16].

By mimicking the action of estrogen, BPA can cause some modifications such as benign lesions, endometrial hyperplasia, development of ovarian cysts and increase in the ductile density of the mammary glands. Regarding the pituitary gland functions, BPA disrupts the production and secretion of gonadotropin-releasing hormones (GnRH) from the hypothalamus and this in turn would also affect the production of the gonadotropins (LH and FSH) from the pituitary gland. Due to the importance of gonadotropins on the function of the gonads, any disruption in their activity can compromise fertility and reproductive health. The reproductive complications of BPA are expressed differently in males and females. In an animal study carried out by [17], where they administered different doses of BPA to male rats at infant and adolescent stages. The results showed that BPA exposure at these stages caused histological alterations and also reduced sperm cells quality and quantity at both stages. Also, there was noticeable alterations in the levels of the sex hormones as levels of LH and FSH were elevated as well as the testosterone levels. Gupta et al. [18] also reviewed studies about BPA exposure and infertility in men. The underlying mechanism of BPA induced pathology is believed to be disruption in the steroidogenesis pathway and increased oxidative stress [19]. There was decreased sperm quality and motility in exposed. Also, low sperm counts, abnormal sperm morphology and elevated FSH levels were shown in a similar study [18]. The ability of BPA to mimic estrogen sometimes allows it to bind to estrogen receptors in the brain and this would lead to alterations in the feedback system which can disrupt the release of hormones. However, in the hypothalamo-pituitary-ovarian axis, it causes a series of changes that develop into symptoms that are related to infertility. This has been proven by both animal and human studies. In animal studies carried out by [20], they examined the effect of BPA exposure in adolescent rats and their experiments revealed that exposure of these newborn rats caused some alteration in their hormone profile as well as some histological changes that were peculiar with a common endocrine disorder in women known as polycystic ovarian syndrome (PCOS). It was noticed that the serum level of FSH and LH were elevated, this is a hallmark of PCOS in females. Also there was presence of multiple defective follicles in the histomorphometry of the ovaries. This observation was also made by [21] on the effects of BPA on ovaries of exposed rats. These degenerative changes were caused by BPA's interference with folliculogenesis. Also in reference to PCOS, another major symptom which is hyperandrogenism was noticed in the serum analysis of the exposed rats as the level of testosterone was markedly increased. In human studies, there was reported irregularities in the menstrual cycle and also the development of PCOS which could both lead to infertility [18]. Due to the sensitivity of the female menstrual cycle and fertility to hormonal imbalances and alteration in endocrine function, it can be established that BPA and other endocrine disruptors can have an adverse effect on the reproductive health of individuals. Whilst BPA is very common in our environment nowadays, it is imperative that some lifestyle amendments are made to reduce interaction and exposure to BPA such as:

- The use of BPA-free products: People should actively look out for "BPA-free" labeled products when shopping for water bottles, food containers and other plastic products that may contain BPA.

- Eating fresh foods: Materials used in processing and packaging processed food may be containing BPA and instead people should opt for fresh foods, frozen foods and vegetables.

- Using glass or stainless steel containers for food storage instead of plastics.

- Avoiding thermal paper receipts whenever possible because they are often BPA-coated.

4.2.1 Polycystic ovarian syndrome

In females, a major disorder of the HPG axis is polycystic ovarian syndrome (PCOS). It is the most common endocrine disorder that occurs in women of reproductive age, affecting a reported 6–10% of adolescents and adult women [22]. PCOS is characterized by the development of multiple cysts on the ovaries and is accompanied by some hallmark symptoms like menstrual cycle abnormalities and hyperandrogenemia (abnormally high level of male sex hormones). LH stimulates the theca cells in the ovaries to produce androgens, these androgens are converted into estrogen by the action of an enzyme known as aromatase. In HPG dysfunction, the androgen is not converted into estrogen and this leads to the hyperandrogenemia. This leads to an array of symptoms that include hirsutism, acne, polycystic ovaries and usually menstrual abnormalities with infertility. Our study has shown that environmental toxins such as bisphenol-A causes hyperandrogenaemia, as shown by increase in the luteinizing hormone of the pituitary and consequently in the testosterone level. These hyperandrogenic states demonstrated poses risks similar to those seen in PCOS states, which can result in anovulation and consequent conception difficulties.

5. Conclusion

The importance of the pituitary gland in fertility preservation and reproduction cannot be understated because it secretes the hormones that stimulate the gonads to produce the sex hormones required for reproduction. The gonadotropins secreted by the pituitary are also necessary for sex cell development, i.e. spermatogenesis and oogenesis. Deficiencies of the pituitary gland and HPG axis that are concerned with hormone imbalances can be as a result of insufficiency of the specific organ (testes or ovary) or problems from the hypothalamus or pituitary gland that affect these organs. These disorders are majorly attributed to insufficient or excessive hormones resulting in complication such as infertility. Diagnosis of these disorders includes measuring the basal hormone levels in the serum. These disorders can be managed through means of medications, hormone replacement therapy or even surgery depending on the severity it poses. Recent upsurge in exposure to endocrine disrupting chemicals (Bisphenol-A inclusive) will in future culminate into increased incidence of pituitary reproductive hormonal imbalances, thereby distorting the gonadal milieu with concurrent rise in fertility issues.

Author details

Eniola Risikat Kadir[1*], Abdulmalik Omogbolahan Hussein[1], Lekan Sheriff Ojulari[2] and Gabriel O. Omotoso[1]

1 Department of Anatomy, College of Health Sciences, University of Ilorin, Ilorin, Nigeria

2 Department of Physiology, College of Health Sciences, University of Ilorin, Ilorin, Nigeria

*Address all correspondence to: kadir.re@unilorin.edu.ng

References

[1] Gounden V, Rampursat YD, Jialal I. Secretory tumors of the pituitary gland: A clinical biochemistry perspective. Clinical Chemistry and Laboratory Medicine. 2018;**57**(2):150-164. DOI: 10.1515/cclm-2018-0552

[2] Melmed S. Pituitary-tumor endocrinopathies. The New England Journal of Medicine. 2020;**382**(10): 937-950. DOI: 10.1056/NEJMra1810772

[3] Melmed S. Pathogenesis of pituitary tumors. Nature Reviews. Endocrinology. 2011;**7**(5):257-266. DOI: 10.1038/nrendo.2011.40

[4] Charitou MM, Mathew R. A case of exaggerated pituitary hyperplasia in a pregnant woman. JCEM Case Reports. 2023;**1**(1). DOI: 10.1210/jcemcr/luad003. Available from: https://academic.oup.com/jcemcr/article/1/1/luad003/7025469

[5] Rawindraraj AD, Basit H, Jialal I. Physiology, anterior pituitary. In: StatPearls. StatPearls Publishing; 2022

[6] Nedresky D, Singh G. Physiology, luteinizing hormone. In: StatPearls. StatPearls Publishing; 2022

[7] Elsherbiny A, Tricomi M, Bhatt D, Dandapantula HK. State-of-the-art: A review of cardiovascular effects of testosterone replacement therapy in adult males. Current Cardiology Reports. 2017;**19**(4):35. DOI: 10.1007/s11886-017-0838-x

[8] Popat VB, Prodanov T, Calis KA, Nelson LM. The menstrual cycle: A biological marker of general health in adolescents. Annals of the New York Academy of Sciences. 2008;**1135**:43-51. DOI: 10.1196/annals.1429.040

[9] WHO. (2012). State of Science of Endocrine Disrupting Chemicals. United Nations Environment Program and the World Health Organization. Inter-Organization Program for the Sound Management of Chemicals. ISBN: 978-92-807-3274-0.

[10] Abraham A, Chakraborty P. A review on sources and health impacts of bisphenol a. Reviews on Environmental Health. 2020;**35**(2):201-210. DOI: 10.1515/reveh-2019-0034

[11] Kawa IA, Masood A, Fatima Q, Mir SA, Jeelani H, Manzoor S, et al. Endocrine disrupting chemical bisphenol A and its potential effects on female health. Diabetes & Metabolic Syndrome. 2021;**15**(3):803-811. DOI: 10.1016/j.dsx.2021.03.031

[12] Rolfo A, Nuzzo AM, De Amicis R, Moretti L, Bertoli S, Leone A. Fetal-maternal exposure to endocrine disruptors: Correlation with diet intake and pregnancy outcomes. Nutrients. 2020;**12**(6):1744. DOI: 10.3390/nu12061744

[13] Thent ZC, Froemming GRA, Ismail ABM, Fuad SBSA, Muid S. Phytoestrogens by inhibiting the non-classical oestrogen receptor, overcome the adverse effect of bisphenol A on hFOB 1.19 cells. Iranian Journal of Basic Medical Sciences. 2020;**23**(9):1155-1163. DOI: 10.22038/ijbms.2020.45296.10545

[14] Dumitrascu MC, Mares C, Petca RC, Sandru F, Popescu RI, Mehedintu C, et al. Carcinogenic effects of bisphenol A in breast and ovarian cancers. Oncology Letters. 2020;**20**(6):282. DOI: 10.3892/ol.2020.12145

[15] Rubin BS, Lenkowski JR, Schaeberle CM, Vandenberg LN,

Ronsheim PM, Soto AM. Evidence of altered brain sexual differentiation in mice exposed perinatally to low, environmentally relevant levels of bisphenol A. Endocrinology. 2006;**147**(8):3681-3691. DOI: 10.1210/en.2006-0189

[16] Lang IA, Galloway TS, Scarlett A, Henley WE, Depledge M, Wallace RB. Association of urinary bisphenol a concentration with medical disorders and laboratory abnormalities in adults. JAMA. 2008;**300**(11):1303-1310. DOI: 10.1001/jama.300.11.1303

[17] Kadir ER, Ojulari LS, Gegele TA, Lawal IA, Sulu-Gambari L, Sulaimon FA, et al. Altered testicular Histomorphometric and antioxidant levels following In vivo bisphenol-a administration. Iranian Journal of Toxicology. 2021;**15**(3):165-174. DOI: 10.32598/IJT.15.3.796.1

[18] Gupta P, Mahapatra A, Suman A, Kumar Singh R. Effect of endocrine disrupting chemicals on HPG Axis: A reproductive endocrine homeostasis. In: Hot Topics in Endocrinology and Metabolism. London, UK, Rijeka: IntechOpen; 2021. DOI: 10.5772/intechopen.96330

[19] Quan C, Wang C, Duan P, Huang W, Chen W, Tang S, et al. Bisphenol a induces autophagy and apoptosis concurrently involving the Akt/mTOR pathway in testes of pubertal SD rats. Environmental Toxicology. 2017;**32**(8):1977-1989. DOI: 10.1002/tox.22339

[20] Kadir ER, Imam A, Olajide OJ, Ajao MS. Alterations of Kiss 1 receptor, GnRH receptor and nuclear receptors of the hypothalamo-pituitary-ovarian axis following low dose of bisphenol-A exposure in Wistar rats. Anatomy & Cell Biology. 2021;**54**:212-224

[21] Aydın V, Ömeroğlu S, Kartal B, Coşkun-akçay N, Akarca-dizakar SÖ, Türkoğlu İ, et al. The effects of antioxidant melatonin on rat ovary neonatal exposure to bisphenol A. Duzce Medical Journal. 2018;**19**(2):33-37

[22] Mikhael S, Punjala-Patel A, Gavrilova-Jordan L. Hypothalamo-pituitary-ovarian axis disorders impacting female fertility. Biomedicine. 2019;**7**(1):5. DOI: 10.3390/biomedicines7010005

Section 4

Complementary Therapies for Pituitary Stimulation

Chapter 5

Perspective Chapter: Stimulation and Activation of the Pituitary Gland

Nilima Dongre

Abstract

The pituitary gland no larger than a pea in shape is located at the base of the brain and is called the "master" gland of the endocrine system because it controls the functions of many other endocrine glands including thyroid, parathyroid, pancreas, reproductive, and adrenal gland. The pituitary gland is attached to the hypothalamus (a part of the brain that affects the pituitary gland) by nerve fibers and blood vessels. The pituitary gland regulates the hormones that have to do with growth, digestion, protein absorption, use, and controlling blood pressure. Overactivity and underactivity of this pea-sized gland on the skull base of the brain can cause a various range of disorders. Since pituitary gland and hypothalamus work together so closely that if one of them is damaged, it can affect the hormonal function of the other. Endocrinologists treat the issues related to the abnormal functioning of this gland by therapeutic interventions. Now-a–days, the concept of mindfulness is widely accepted to treat endocrine disorders. Psychoneuroendocrinology is the new upcoming branch in therapeutics of several neuroendocrine diseases. The pituitary gland disorders can also be corrected by lifestyle modifications like practicing certain yoga asanas, pranayama, and meditations.

Keywords: psychoneuroendocrinology, lifestyle modifications, yoga asanas, pranayama, meditation

1. Introduction: the pituitary gland

A small pea-shaped pituitary gland is referred to as the body's master gland as it controls many vital body functions via controlling the activity of most other hormone-secreting glands including thyroid, parathyroid, pancreas, reproductive, and adrenal gland. It plays a major role in regulating vital body functions and general well-being.

Anatomically, the pituitary gland is like a protrusion at the base of the brain and the size of this is a pea or cherry. The gland is located in a well-protected small bony cavity sella turcica of the skull, level with the eyes, and roughly in the middle of the head.

It is attached to the hypothalamus of the brain which controls the involuntary (vegetative) nervous system. This part of nervous system helps in managing the activities like balance of energy, heat and water including body temperature, heartbeat, urination, sleep, hunger, and thirst. The gland also produces several hormones which regulate most of the hormone-producing glands in the body or have a direct effect on the target organs especially thyroid, reproductive organs, adrenal gland etc. [1, 2]. This hormone secretion generates inhibitory or stimulatory signals from the hypothalamus.

The pituitary gland can be divided into two lobes: Anterior pituitary lobe and Posterior pituitary lobe.

1.1 Anterior pituitary lobe

It is made of several different types of cells which produce and releases the following different types of hormones:

1. Growth hormone (GH): This hormone regulates growth and physical development. Primary targets of this hormone are bone and muscles. It can also stimulate growth in almost all tissues of the body.

2. Thyroid-stimulating hormone (TSH): This thyroid-stimulating hormone which activates the thyroid to release the thyroid hormones are very crucial in controlling the overall metabolism.

3. Adrenocorticotropic hormone (ACTH): This hormone stimulates the adrenal gland for the production of cortisol and other hormones.

4. Follicle-stimulating hormones: This hormone is involved in the secretion of estrogen and the growth of ovum in women and sperm cell production in men.

5. Luteinizing hormone (LH):This hormone is involved in the production of the sex hormones like estrogen in women and testosterone in men.

6. Prolactin helps in the production of milk in breastfeeding women.

7. Endorphins have pain-relieving properties and are thought to be connected to the pleasure centers of the brain.

8. Enkephalins are closely related to endorphins and also have pain-relieving effects.

9. Beta-melanocyte-stimulating hormone: This hormone stimulates increased pigmentation in response to exposure to UV radiation.

1.2 Posterior pituitary lobe

This section of the pituitary gland also secretes hormones—vasopressin and oxytocin. These hormones are usually produced in the hypothalamus and stored in the posterior lobe till they are released.

Vasopressin: This hormone is also called as antidiuretic hormone. It helps body in water conservation and prevents dehydration.

Oxytocin: This hormone stimulates the release of breast milk and helps in contractions of uterus during labor [1, 2].

The disorders of the pituitary gland are pituitary tumors, hypopituitarism, Cushing's syndrome, acromegaly, hyperprolactinemia, and diabetes insipidus and disorder due to traumatic injury to the brain.

Following are the common symptoms seen in the disorders of the pituitary gland: headaches, generalized weakness or fatigue, unexplained weight gain, high blood pressure, insomnia, mood swings, psychological state changes, depression, memory loss, reproductive issues like infertility, erectile dysfunctions and irregular menses, excessive or unusual hair growth, and lactation is found when the individual is not nursing.

2. Hypothalamus pituitary axis

The three components, the hypothalamus, the pituitary gland, and the adrenal glands comprise the HPA axis or HPTA axis. This HPA axis represents a complex set of direct influences and feedback interactions among them.

This HPA axis is a major neuroendocrine system that has control over the reactions to stress and other various major body processes like digestion, immunity, moods and emotions, sexuality, energy storage, and expenditure. It serves as a common mechanism for interactions among glands, hormones, and part of the midbrain [3, 4]. As steroid hormones are produced in the vertebrates, there is a direct link between the HPA axis and corticosteroids under stress.

The functioning of the HPA axis is affected by various factors including exposure to early life stress situations. These affect the brain's endocrine system and will suppress the neuronal responses and immunity of an individual. Chronic stress leads to an increase in cortisol release. Too much cortisol release can sometimes lead to insomnia, weight gain, anxiety, and depression.

This will affect the quality of an individual's behavior throughout the life. Treatment of such chronic life situations with drug therapy is routinely practiced by endocrinologists. In the long run, they show side effects.

Recently, alternative therapies are proven to be better in the treatment of the chronic diseases. These alternative therapies work on the holistic approach—they are noninvasive and are with less side effects.

3. Mind–body disease interactions

The studies in infant development and neuroscience are proving the modern developments in psychoanalytical theory to produce a coherent link between mind–body diseases. The studies reported that the infant's failure to environmental responses leads to fragile vulnerable personality structure that relies on external objects to regulate psychobiological responses. These responses are mediated through the rostral limbic system and expressed through changes in the HPA axis and autonomic nervous system. The article written by John Mason (1968) concluded that as a perception of stressful situation, the novelty, unpredictability, high ego involvement, anticipation on negative consequences, and uncontrollability are the behaviors exhibited by an individual. The HPA axis regulates and controls the overall psychological and neurological behaviors of an individual.

4. Yoga and pituitary health

The Bhagwad Gita—quotes "Yoga is the Journey of the self Through the Self, To the Self." In the Indian scriptures, yoga and yogic science have proven to be effective tools for the overall health and wellbeing of an individual.

"Yoga is a complete science of Ancient Indian system of Medicine which is more than 5000 years old whereas the present more prevalent system of allopathic medicine is nearly 200 years old only" [5].

As the body's biochemistry starts changing from the age of 20 years, it is advised that practicing some yoga for at least half an hour everyday will keep the body's biochemistry fit and help us to be healthy [6].

Yoga helps in the following ways to improve our health:

1. Improves flexibility
2. Helps build muscle strength
3. Helps in perfecting your posture
4. Reduces cartilage and joint breakdown
5. Protects your spine
6. Improves bone health
7. Increases blood circulation
8. Drains lymph and upsurges immunity
9. Increases heart rate
10. Reduces blood pressure
11. Regulates the adrenal gland function
12. Makes you feel happy
13. Gives you a healthy life style
14. Reduces blood sugar
15. Relaxes body systems
16. Increases focus and concentration
17. Maintains the nervous system
18. Releases the tension in limbs
19. Improves sleep quality
20. Increase self esteem

4.1 Yoga and pituitary health

Practicing yoga regularly helps us to achieve complete physical and mental health scientifically. Yoga is also emerging as a more effective way of nonpharmacological and noninvasive endocrine therapy against many diseases including the pituitary health. A complete physical and mental wellbeing state can only be achieved by following healthy lifestyles, healthy eating habits, maintaining physical fitness together with maintaining spiritual and emotional health. Yogic way of living helps to achieve optimum physical, mental, and spiritual health. Several studies have reported that yoga helps in achieving health through its influence on the endocrine system of our body. Endocrine system hormones are the primary messengers that are produced by several endocrine glands, i.e., hypothalamus, pituitary gland, adrenal glands, thyroid gland, parathyroid glands, pancreas, and gonads of the body. The exact meaning of the term "endocrine" means a process of specific stimuli causing the release of the hormones from the glands into the bloodstream. For a balanced hormonal function in all the changing environment, it is necessary that all the hormonal systems in the body function in a synchronous manner and regulate each other. Many releasing hormones are secreted by hypothalamus in the brain and are transmitted to the pituitary gland via blood circulation. The major role of these releasing hormones is induction and controlling of the secretion of the pituitary hormones which in turn are transported via blood to various target hormonal glands of the body. The feedback from these target glands to the hypothalamus and pituitary controls the further release and maintain the hormonal balance. These feedbacks cause a negative and or positive effect on hormone production.

5. The lifestyle modifications and pituitary gland

The hormonal change in both men and women significantly impacts the quality of life. It is found that the hormonal imbalance affects the cognitive function, i.e., ability to think or analyze. These also cause issues like bloating, headaches, sleep disturbances, eating disorders, weight gain, skin issues, and lowering immunity, and many more even on small changes in the hormonal imbalances. If not properly diagnosed at the early stages, this may lead to several chronic diseases [7].

A significant health challenge is the emergence of stress and stress-related diseases. According to the traditional definition of stress, it is the real or predicted disruption of homeostasis caused by particular physical and emotional occurrences known as "stressors." A damaging, self-replicating cascade of neuroendocrine, metabolic, and cognitive abnormalities brought on by protracted exposure to stress can be crucial in the onset and development of cardiovascular disease (CVD), such as hypertension.

The HPA axis and the sympathoadrenal system (SAS), which consists of the sympathetic nervous system (SNS) and adrenomedullary system (AS), are the two components of complex stress system that mediates the body's reactions to stressors. The main mediators of the stress response are the hormones of the HPA axis and the catecholamines generated by SAS.

The paraventricular nucleus of the hypothalamus, or PVN, is a key component in the stress response. The production of CRH and Arginine vasopressin (AVP), which starts the endocrine response to stressors, is caused by stress-induced activation of the parvocellular neurons of the PVN. The anterior pituitary gland's ability to secrete ACTH is governed by CRH. In PVN parvocellular neurons, AVP colocalizes with CRH. AVP amplifies the result of in the anterior pituitary.

AVP increases the impact of CRH on ACTH release in the anterior pituitary. The noradrenergic neurons in the locus ceruleus (LC) and CRH neurons in the PVN have reciprocal connections, which causes them to stimulate one another in a positive feedback manner. The adrenocortical and autonomic branches of the stress response are connected by CRH, which functions as a neurotransmitter that mediates sympathetic arousal. The sympathetic nervous systems (SNS) stimulation in response to stress is regulated by the locus ceruleus-norepinephrine system (LNE). Glucocorticoid production from the adrenal cortex is primarily regulated by ACTH. The HPA axis, which regulates how an organism reacts to stimuli, is final affected by glucocorticoid chemicals, primarily cortisol in humans and cortisone in animals.

During the initial phase of the acute stress response, the SAS is engaged, resulting in the typical "fight-or-flight" behaviors. These are rapid but transient physiological adjustments made to get ready for the challenge posed by a stressful event. It is mediated by the release of catecholamine like norepinephrine (NE). The secondary phase involves a hormonal mechanism (HPA axis) that is thought to be slower than the synaptic mechanisms that activate the SAS, but which nonetheless causes an amplified and prolonged secretory response involving stress hormones like CRH, ACTH, and glucocorticoids (GCs), with cortisol being the main GC involved in humans (long-lasting response). Cortisol has an impact on the brain as well as other bodily components.

The body's capacity to process stresses cognitively and physically is further hampered by stress-induced brain alterations. Multiple interconnected organ systems (autonomic, neuroendocrine, immune, and cardiovascular systems) involved in the stress response are negatively impacted by the prolonged and synergistic effects of stress hormones and pro-inflammatory cytokines in chronic stress, which ultimately leads to various pathological conditions [8].

There are several simple ways to take care of the pituitary gland and its functioning, which are as follows:

1. Wake up early in the morning
2. Eat proper and nutritious food,
3. Practice yoga and meditation to reduce stress
4. Get good quality sleep
5. Withdrawal from addictions like smoking tobacco and alcoholism
6. Take care about the consumption of food toxins and adulterants
7. Regular physical activity
8. Keep away from sugars and other food allergens
9. Add lots of fiber and good-quality protein in diet
10. Consume healthy fats.

Several studies have indicated that frequent yoga practice is linked to decreased basal cortisol and catecholamine release, decreased sympathetic activity, and increased parasympathetic activity. It is supposed to result from yoga's ability to reduce stress. Yoga's ability to reduce stress may be a result of modulating limbic signals, which, through the hypothalamus, can change sympathetic activity and the hormone response to stress. In addition to helping to reduce cortisol levels and alleviate stress, yoga may also increase hippocampus 5HT1A receptor activity [9–11].

Gamma-aminobutyric acid (GABA) mediates the amplitude and duration of the stress response and thus negatively regulates excitability in the PVN. This leads to direct inhibition of HPA axis. Yoga modulates this GABA-nergic stimulation of HPA axis. Regular yogic practices have shown to increase the GABA levels in the thalamus. This may be attributed to the ability of yoga practices to increase in the activity of parasympathetic nervous system [12–17].

Yoga mediates downregulation of HPA axis and sympathoadrenal system, stimulation of vagus resulting in parasympathetic dominance, increase in baroreflex sensitivity, and increase in brain GABA levels inhibiting PVN integrating area of stress signals. Thus, mediates the beneficial effects on overall health of an individual.

6. Conclusion

This chapter mainly focuses on the alternative ways of stimulating and activating the pituitary gland and maintaining the hormonal balance in the body by alternative noninvasive ways of medicine like practicing yoga and adopting healthy lifestyle practices. Yogic intervention modifies neuro-endocrine modulation of the stress response and exerts its positive benefits via a number of distinct mechanisms. Yoga reduces the neuro-humoral reaction to stress. Proper mind–body interactions are very important in an individual to have a healthy life. Yogic practices help in achieving them. A contented and mindful life is the key for a healthy life in this modern technological /mechanical era.

Conflict of interest

The author declares she has no conflict of interest.

Author details

Nilima Dongre
BLDE (DU) Shri B.M. Patil Medical College, Hospital and Research Centre, Vijayapura, Karnataka, India

*Address all correspondence to: nilima.donge@bldedu.ac.in

References

[1] Health Info/Hormones Pituitary Gland Disorders – Signs, Symptoms, Treatments. Last Updated by Dr. Gurvinder Rull, Peer Reviewed by Dr. Adrian Bonsall. Last Updated 28 Sep 2018

[2] Pituitary Gland: Anatomy, Function, Diagram, Conditions. Healthline. Availabe from: https://www.healthline.com>human-body-maps>pit. 11 Jun 2018-Pituitary Gland Overview, Medically Reviewed by Suzanne Falck, By Jill Seladi-Schulman- Updated on June 11, 2018

[3] Malenka RC, Nestler EJ, Hymen SE. Chapter10: Neural and neuroendocrine control of Internal Milieu. In: Sydor A, Brown RY, editors. Neuropharmacology: A Foundation for Clinical Neuroscience. 2nd ed. New York: McGraw Hill Medical; 2009. pp. 248-259

[4] Hans S. Stress without Distress. Philadelphia: Lippincott; 1974

[5] Read NW. Chapter 30 - Bridging the gap between mind and body: Do cultural and psychoanalytic concepts of visceral disease have an explanation in contemporary neuroscience? In: Mayer EA, Saper CB, editors. Progress in Brain Research. Vol. 122. London, UK: Elsevier; 2000. pp. 425-443. DOI: 10.1016/S0079-6123(08)62155-X. Available from: https://www.sciencedirect.com/science/article/pii/S007961230862155X

[6] Singh SP. Biochemistry: The 'Yoga' and the 'Health' in Textbook of Biochemistry. 6th ed. Darya Gunj, New Delhi: CBS Publishers & Distributors PVT Ltd; 2015. pp. 983-984

[7] Enkhmaa B, Surampudi P, Anuurad E, et al. Lifestyle changes: Effect of diet, exercise, functional food, and obesity treatment on lipids and lipoproteins. In: Feingold KR, Anawalt B, Blackman MR, et al., editors. Endotext. South Dartmouth (MA): MDText.com, Inc.; 2000. Available from: https://www.ncbi.nlm.nih.gov/books/NBK326737/

[8] Shripati WS. Stress, Hypertension and Yoga: Effects of Stress on Human Health. London, UK: IntechOpen; 2020. DOI: 10.5772/Intechopen.88147

[9] Kyizom T, Singh S, Singh KP, Tandon OP, Kumar R. Effect of pranayama & yoga-asana on cognitive brain functions in type 2 diabetes-P3 event related evoked potential (ERP). Indian Journal of Medical Research. 2010;**131**:636-640

[10] Parshad O. Role of yoga in stress management. West Indian Medical Journal. 2005;**11**:711-717

[11] Gupta N, Khera S, Vempati RP, Sharma R, Bijlani RL. Effect of yoga based lifestyle intervention on state and trait anxiety. Indian Journal of Physiology & Pharmacology. 2006;**50**:41-47

[12] Kovacs KJ, Miklos IH, Bali B. GABAergic mechanisms constraining the activity of the hypothalamopituitary-adrenocortical axis. Annals of New York Academy of Sciences. 2004;**1018**:466-476

[13] Jessop DS, Renshaw D, Larsen PJ, Chowdrey HS, Harbuz MS. Substance P is involved in terminating the hypothalamo-pituitary-adrenal axis response to acute stress through centrally located neurokinin-1 receptors. Stress. 2000;**3**:209-220

[14] Li DP, Pan HL. Role of gammaaminobutyric acid (GABA)a and

(GABA)B receptors in paraventricular nucleus in control of sympathetic vasomotor tone in hypertension. The Journal of Pharmacology and Expermental Therapeutics. 2007;**320**(2):615-626

[15] Streeter CC, Whitfield TH, Owen L, Rein T, Karri SK, Yakhkind A, et al. Effects of yoga versus walking on mood, anxiety, and brain GABA levels: A randomized controlled MRS study. The Journal of Alternative and Complementary Medicine. 2010;**16**(11):1145-1152

[16] Lee MS, Huh HJ, Kim BG, et al. Effects of qi-training on heart rate variability. The American Journal of Chinese Medicine. 2002;**30**:463-470

[17] Radley JJ, Sawchenko PE. A common substrate for prefrontal and hippocampal inhibition of the neuroendocrine stress response. The Journal of Neuroscience. 2011;**31**(26):9683-9969